# ESSENTIAL OILS

# ESSENTIAL OILS

## A Concise Manual of Their Therapeutic Use in Herbal and Aromatic Medicine

*Nikki Darrell*

**AEON**

First edition published in 2022 by
Aeon Books

British Library Cataloguing in Publication Data

A C.I.P. for this book is available from the British Library

ISBN-13: 978-1-80152-016-4

Typeset by Medlar Publishing Solutions Pvt Ltd, India

www.aeonbooks.co.uk

# CONTENTS

CHAPTER 9
**It's all about the base-carrier oils, macerated oils, and creams**         125

# *INTRODUCTION*

This is a concise manual to help practitioners to include essential oils in their therapeutic repertoire. Drawing on my experience as a practitioner, this book is the culmination of more than thirty years of using essential oils for their amazing capacity to promote health.

Here, I focus on the essential oils that have a broader range of use, are safe to use in general practice, and are generally affordable and accessible.

We will start be exploring the nature of essential oils, the importance of quality, and how to blend them. Then, moving onto some specific profiles, we shall finally look at the use of essential oils for different conditions and some formulations that I have found particularly valuable.

Since I first started working with essential oils, there have been many changes in how essential oils are marketed and an increase in multilevel marketing (MLM) companies promoting their use intensively and internally without any level of clinical training. In my experience, the times that internal use is needed are few and far between; delivering them through the skin and by inhalation is safer and often yields better results. Intensive use has its place, but let's remember that essential oils are extremely concentrated and with a significant number of them, less is more. It is always wise to err on the side of safe practice, and it is also more economical to use oils in smaller amounts.

As the use of essential oils becomes more popular we also need to consider sustainable and ethical sourcing. With all the plants we use, we need to ask whether their production and harvest is good for the ecosystem they are coming from, and whether those who cultivate, harvest, and distil the plants are receiving a fair price for their produce. By ensuring we responsibly source the essential oils we use, we support social, economical, and environmental sustainability within this sector. These are important issues to explore, which we can address by working with suppliers who follow these ethics and can readily supply accurate information about where they are sourcing.

I first trained in Holistic Aromatherapy in the late eighties, studying with Patricia Davis at the London School of Aromatherapy. From there, I trained with Shirley Price in Clinical Aromatherapy and then in Aromatic Medicine with Daniel Penoel, a French doctor specialising in the use of essential oils in his practice; there is a long history of the use of essential oils as medicine in France.

The expanse of therapeutic applications of essential oils opened up to me and was complemented by my work alongside a herbalist who had learned much of his approach from his grandfather. In their practice the use of essential oils in some formulations and preparations was an intrinsic aspect of herbalism. At herbal college, I was surprised that the use of aromatherapy and essential oils were rather frowned upon, and considered to be a fanciful indulgence from the world of beauty therapy rather than a serious and valid part of plant medicine, which stood in sharp contrast to Dr Penoel's work as a doctor.

At that time, there were some small specialist companies supplying excellent quality oils to the therapeutic sector. Larger companies, however, supplied the food and fragrance industry, but these oils were adjusted and sometimes adulterated, rather than being complete oils obtained by distillation from single botanical species; in these sectors the interest was in oils that gave consistent taste or fragrance rather than the full complex oils.

It is generally agreed amongst those who have been working with essential oils over the past few decades that the best quality oils are produced by small scale artisan producers. Those who have learned their skill over years of practice and use the best quality plant material often harvest by hand and at the optimum time for the best quality oil to be extracted. There is great diversity in the scent and composition of a true essential oil, depending upon the season and region it comes from—they should not be homogenous in nature.

There are so many different essential oils available and I have not included them all in the profiles but selected the ones I feel are most useful and therefore worth investing in. My collection includes about 60–80 different oils, but they are such a major part of my practice. An awareness of the environmental impact of our medicine is crucial—as healers it is our duty to protect the environment and the nature that is the foundation of our practice. We can also help educate the wider public about the need to care for our ecosystems and how to responsibly engage in herbal medicine. For example, when Helichrysum rose to 'fame' the wild population in Croatia was severely overharvested and thankfully it has now recovered, but this took over five years.

Although I will allude to some aromatic waters and fixed/carrier oils in the formulae section, these are both large sections of our materia medica deserving of their own books, so I have not included large amounts of material about them in the text.

Personally, I have seen that the use of these highly concentrated extracts of plants and the topical or transdermal application of herbs to be a most valuable and underused way of working for many herbalists. There are many ways of integrating essential oils into your practice, and this is just a small tome sharing the ways I have found effective.

# CHAPTER 1

# The nature of essential oils

E ssential oils are complex mixtures of substances, produced by distillation from a single botanical species. They may contain up to 350 different molecules, some of which have been closely studied, some of which have yet to be identified. True essential oils are only produced by distillation, and differ from the essence directly produced in the plant in that some of the constituents will be altered in the process. If the process is carried out correctly, this can enhance the therapeutic value of the essential oil; chamazulene is produced during the distillation of German Chamomile and is a very important anti-inflammatory substance with a deep blue colour, which is not present in the herb. Conversely, bad distillation can cause the production of undesirable components, such as skin irritant molecules in terpene rich oils.

Some practitioners also use essences, produced by cold expression.

There is a certain amount of controversy over whether only oils from organically grown crops should be used, due to the potential carry over of pesticides and herbicides from conventionally grown plants. However, it should be noted that many growers do not use artificial chemicals or pesticides, but are not organically certified due to the cost of certification. Also, it is possible to get organically produced oils of variable quality, so it is best to deal with suppliers you know get well-produced oils. It is best to try out different products and decide what you are happy to work with and what you can afford to work with. Just remember, the better the quality of your oils, the more effective they will be and that a bad oil will do no favours to anyone.

We will examine the processes of oil production, storage, and purity further on, but first we will look at the general character of the essential oils.

Essential oils differ from 'fixed' oils in that they are not greasy. They are volatile substances (otherwise they couldn't be distilled!) of an essentially polar nature, which means they are mainly insoluble in water, but will dissolve readily in fats, oils, waxes, and organic solvents, including ethanol. Being volatile, they must be stored in closed containers, and recovered after dispensing, otherwise they will evaporate. Also, exposure to oxygen in the air can cause chemical reactions known as oxidation to occur, giving rise to break down products. This also means that small amounts should not be left in large bottles, but should be decanted into a smaller one. Their solubility in alcohol is limited, and some components have a limited solubility in water, which is why hydrolats (also known as hydrosols or aromatic waters) have an aroma. All essential oils have an aroma, which may be perceived as more or less pleasant. They may be virtually colourless, varying shades of yellow and brown,, whilst some are brightly coloured; German Chamomile is dark blue, Bergamot is a shade of green, whilst Reunion Geranium is a different green hue. Cold pressed Lemon is a rich yellow, and Patchouli is deep brown. Due to the fact that essential oils are made up of organic compounds (ones containing carbon and hydrogen), they can dissolve certain synthetic materials, including plastic and some varnishes; they should always be stored in glass. It also means that essential oils should not be spilled on varnished or polished surfaces, as they will mark them.

## The extraction of essential oils

### Distillation

The only method that produces true essential oils. The plant tissue is placed in a deep vat and steam is passed through it. The steam that passes through picks up molecules with an atomic weight lower than

300, and larger components such as tannins and bitters are too heavy to carry over in the steam so are left behind.

The vaporised water and essential oils are collected by cooling through a water column, the essential oils are separated off and the water phase is passed through the still several times to saturate it with volatile components and then decanted and stored to be used therapeutically as a hydrosol. Distillation is a highly technical process and a great art, which normally takes a long time to master. If the distiller is inexperienced, the oil may of little or no therapeutic value. You do not need to understand the process in great depth, but it is important to understand some of the basic principles and the factors that affect its success and quality. There are several types of distillation used to produce essential oils. Water distillation means that the plant material is placed into the still with the water and is gradually heated until the water boils and evaporates. With steam distillation super-heated steam is introduced into the still and travels through the plant material, releasing the volatile components. This method uses much less water, and gives higher yields. A third method is water and steam distillation, where the plant is placed into the still with water, but live steam is generated in a separate chamber and introduced to the main chamber.

Other factors that affect the quality of the essential oil produced are:

**Pressure**—if the chamber is slightly depressurised, so that the pressure is lower than atmospheric pressure, it is possible to distil at a lower temperature. This means than more of the lower volatility components are preserved, as are those which are more heat sensitive. It is less likely that the oil produced will be 'charred' and therefore the quality is far superior.

**Duration**—some components require a longer distillation for extraction. These constituents also tend to have very valuable therapeutic effects and are often more expensive, due to the increased cost of a longer distillation.

**pH**—the acidity of the water used to distil will also affect the final constituents of the oil and it is, therefore, very important to distil each species at the correct pH.

In addition to this, some people would say that the type of material that the still is made from can have a profound effect. For instance, Patchouli from a rusty still is reputed to be of superior quality.

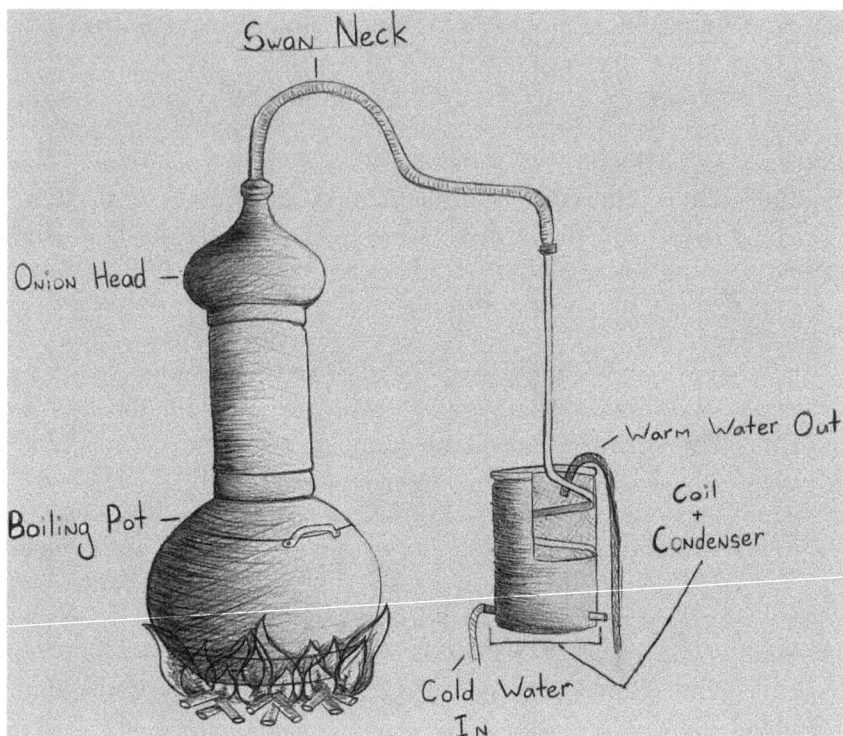

A simple still—Lucy Quane

*Solvent extraction*

This method has largely replaced enfleurage as the method for absolute production. The plant tissue is extracted with hydrocarbon solvents, This method is used for plants that yield small quantities of delicate molecules which may be broken down by the temperatures traditionally used in distillation. Some plants may be distilled or extracted to give either an essential oil or a concrete. Examples are Neroli, Rose (Absolute—extracted or Otto—distilled), and Lavender. Concretes are usually solid, waxy, and more expensive. They are more stable and are used in the perfume industry. Their waxy nature is due to the fact that non-volatile and non-fragrant components, including waxes and pigments, are extracted. They are not suitable for dermal application, since they often contain traces of contaminants. Some resinoids may also be obtained this way. After the initial solvent extraction, the concrete is subjected to a series of alcohol washes to remove waxy residues. A slight heat (about 50°C) is used to remove the last traces of alcohol. This yields an absolute. Absolutes are not recommended for therapeutic use but may be used in individual 'perfume' blends used for their psycho-emotional benefits.

## Enfleurage

This method is virtually never used today, but is the traditional method for extracting some of the most costly essences. Glass plates are coated with a layer of fat or lard and layers of petals are put on top. The volatile substances migrate into the fat, and the petals are removed and replaced until the fat is saturated with the essence. This yields a pomade, which is then treated with alcohol to extract the pure essence.

## Cold pressing or expression

This is the method used to produce essences from the peel of citrus fruit. The rinds are simply squeezed, and the essence is collected in sponges. These are often a by-product of the fruit juice industry. They are the type of citrus oil used in true aromatherapy. Steam distilled essential oils are also produced from the citrus fruits. These are less sensitising to the skin and are mainly used in the food and fragrance industries.

## Aromatic definitions

### Absolute

Originally produced by enfleurage, these are now normally produced by solvent extraction. They are thicker and more viscous than essential oils and contain heavier molecules, sometimes including waxes. Solvent extracted absolutes are not suitable for application to the skin in higher concentrations, and therefore some authorities do not recommend their use in aromatherapy. Enfleurage oils are far more expensive than absolutes (Jasmine can only be produced by these two methods). Oils produced by the enfleurage method are very expensive due to the labour involved and the small yield. Jasmine can only be produced by enfleurage or by solvent extraction. Rose otto (the distilled product) tends to be more expensive than the solvent extract.

## Adulteration

As such high prices can be obtained for some essential oils and aromatic essences, there are many unscrupulous people willing to 'adjust the sauce' (a perfumery term for adulteration!). This may be done in several ways.

The oil may simply be diluted with vegetable oil or alcohol.

Synthetic components may be added to make the profile more appealing to the consumer. This may actually be done before or during distillation. In France, if the Lavender crop in a particular year is low in linalyl acetate (the main fragrance component), it has been known for the plant to be sprayed with synthetic linalyl acetate before distillation.

Alternatively, the essential oil may be partially or totally substituted by a similar smelling oil of lower price and higher yield. Two examples are Melissa and Lemon Verbena. The true oils are at least as expensive as some of the absolutes, but what reaches some outlets is mainly Lemongrass, Citronella, Lemon or Indian Verbena, all of which are very much easier and cheaper to produce.

## Cohobation

The repassing of the water phase through the distillation unit many times to extract as much as possible of the water-soluble aromatic components to prepare hydrosols/aromatic waters.

## Concrete

This is what is extracted from the pomade in traditional enfleurage. As the concrete still contains waxes, it is solid at room temperature and needs further extraction with alcohol to produce an absolute.

## Essential oil

A complex substance, containing a mixture of volatile, organic molecules, extracted from a single botanical species by distillation. Distillation may cause the evolution of valuable components not naturally occurring e.g. chamazulene in German Chamomile (*Chamomilla recutita*). Poor distillation may cause the production of undesirable components e.g. dermal irritants in terpene rich oils. All essential oils are volatile, those with smaller-sized molecules as components being more volatile.

## Hydrosol/hydrolat/floral water/aromatic water

The water phase of the distillation, saturated with water soluble volatile components, such as alcohols and acids. These have their own therapeutic properties and are widely used in many countries both in cooking and as medicines.

N.B. Mixing distilled water and essential oils does not produce the same product. Beware when purchasing these as the synthesised products often contain dispersants, which can irritant delicate skins, rather than being valuable tonics for such. Also, try to obtain those without preservatives, which are also harsh on the skin.

## Rectification (Redistillation)

The essential oil is distilled more than once, either for a shorter time or with one of the other variables altered. This is done to remove specific components. *Rectified oils are not suitable for therapeutic use.* Some oils used in the food, fragrance, or pharmaceutical industries are rectified, whether to remove unwanted components, like terpenes or lower volatility components, or to alter the components in some other way. This is done to give a different fragrance, to remove colour or reduce viscosity.

## Resinoids

Produced from resins (Benzoin, Myrrh, Frankincense) by solvent extraction or distillation. The distilled oils are preferable, as aggressive solvents such as benzene may be used for the solvent extraction.

# CHAPTER 2

# Selecting essential oils and aromatic waters for therapeutic use

E ssential oils, macerated oils, and aromatic waters are produced for use in a range of sectors and it is imperative to use ones of appropriate quality for therapeutic application. When selecting products to use, make sure that they are natural, unadulterated, and follow the guidelines below to ensure that they are. Also, be aware of the supply chain you are using. Your supplier should be able to demonstrate traceability back to the primary producer. The production of gas liquid chromatography (GLC) sheets and so forth are not a guarantee since there is no assurance that the data sheets relate to the batch you are purchasing. So ask your supplier questions—if they are knowledgeable and know what they are selling they will be happy to answer you.

The plant material from which the essential oil is prepared needs to be assessed as regards the following criteria:

### From a single named botanical species

The binomial Latin name for the specific plant species should always be included in the product information. Due to the size of labels which can fit on a 10 ml bottle, this information may not all be on the label, but should be on the price list, and if the supplier cannot answer any questions in this direction, they probably do not understand their products. Knowing the exact plant species is important; for example, *Hyssopus officinalis ssp decumbens* is quite safe even for babies but *Hyssopus officinalis* is neurotoxic, due to its pinocamphone content. *Salvia officinalis* essential oil causes cardiac malformation and malfunction in the foetus. It is also neurotoxic in high doses due to its thujone content. Since it is used to adulterate *Salvia sclarea*, one must be assured of unadulterated oils. *Juniperus communis* and *J. virginiana* are both therapeutically valuable tools, but they have very different actions.

## Country of origin

The crop should be grown in its natural habitat to ensure that the plant produces the secondary metabolites that are therapeutically desirable. Sometimes two oils from different regions can have differing therapeutic properties; Geranium (*Pelargonium graveolens*) from Reunion or Madagascar and from China will be quite different. The oil's constituent profile will be affected by temperature, rain fall, and altitude, amongst other things.

## Part used

This is important to determine. With Juniper, it is the berries that are normally used therapeutically. An oil is also distilled from the branchlets, but this has slightly different properties. With Angelica the seed carries a risk when used on cardiac patients, but the root is ok. With Orange, there are three different oils obtained from the plant-one from the fruit, one from the leaves and one from the flowers.

## Chemotypes

With certain plants such as Thyme, Rosemary, Mint, and Geranium, there can be wide variation in the chemical composition of the oil obtained. Selected clones or cultivars can be cultivated, which are particularly high in certain components. Where the chemotypes are very high in one component, or very low in a toxic or aggressive component, they can be used for very specific therapeutic purposes.

## Harvesting techniques

These should be environmentally friendly, good for the soil and eco-system. For example with lavender when harvesting for the fragrance industry the entire plant is grubbed up which is detrimental to the soil amongst other things. For medicinal use the plants should be hand-picked and re-harvested. Lavender plants can be harvested for up to seven years. On some farms, the spent material from the distillation is returned to the land and sheep are used to plough it in; this really helps enrich the soil and gives back to the plants.

## Correct distillation

In order to get the full range of therapeutic molecules, it is necessary to follow the correct procedure. Low pressure techniques allow the oil to be distilled at lower temperatures, preventing scorching. However, this takes longer and is therefore more expensive. There is a vast difference between such oils and those that are distilled as quickly and incompletely as they are for the fragrance industry. Correct distillation is also important because some of the therapeutic molecules are not present in the plant, only their precursors, therefore if not correctly distilled they will not work! Other components, such as coumarins have a low volatility and require a long distillation time, otherwise they will not be carried over. A high quality *Lavandula officinalis* will contain coumarins, whereas those prepared for the fragrance and food industry will not as they do not contribute to the desired aroma.

## Distilled, not extracted

For clinical use, only oils that have been cold pressed or distilled should be used, including the floral oils.

## Storage

Even if the oils have been grown and distilled correctly, they will not be of therapeutic standard if they are not stored in the correct way. Oils must also be stored in the dark, without contact with the air, at room temperature. Terpene rich oils should be used within one year of extraction, whereas others have a longer shelf life.

## Pure, complete, and natural after distillation

The oil should not be rectified. This means that they should not be redistilled to remove certain components. For example, because terpenes are astringent and quite aggressive in their action, the perfumery industry de-terpenates oils. However, this concentrates other components of the oil.

By following these guidelines when selecting oils, one can ensure that:

- The therapeutic actions can be specified from the chemical profile.
- They are suitable for therapeutic application.
- The purity of the product ensures minimal risk of toxic and allergic reactions in the therapist or patient. With some of the oils that have been assumed to cause reactions, it is because they are adulterated, badly stored, or otherwise treated badly.

# CHAPTER 3

# Safety and contraindications

## Essential oils safe at normal topical dilutions (0–3%)

Benzoin (*Styrax benzoin*), Bergamot (*Citrus bergamia*), Black Pepper (*Piper nigrum*), Chamomile (German/Roman; *Matricaria recutita/Anthemis nobilis*), Cananga (*Cananga odorata*), Citrus (Grapefruit, Lemon, Lime, Mandarin, Orange, Tangerine; *C. aurantium, limomum, reticulata, sinensis, paradisi, tangerina*; petitgrains are essential oils from the citrus plant leaves), Caraway (*Carum carvi*), Cardamom (*Elettaria cardamomum*), Carrot seed (*Daucus carota*), Cedarwood (Atlas, Virginian; *Cedrus atlanica/virginiana*), Citronella, (*Cybopogon nardus/winterianus*), Cinnamon (*Cinnamomum verum*), Clary Sage (*Salvia sclarea*), Clove bud (*Eugenia caryophyllum*), Coriander (*Coriandrum sativum*), Cypress (*Cupressus sempervirens*), Dill (*Anethum graveolens*), Eucalyptuses (*Eucalyptus* spp.), Fennel Sweet (*Foeniculum vulgare*), Frankincense (*Boswellia caterii*), Geranium (*Pelargonium graveolens*), Ginger (*Zingiber officinale*), Helichrysum (*Helichrysum italicum*), Ho Leaf (*Cinnamomum camphora*), Hops (*Humulus lupulus*), Hyssop (*Hyssopus officinalis*), Juniper (*Juniperus communis*), Lavandin (*Lavandula x intermedia*), Lavender (*Lavandula officinalis/angustifolium/vera*), Lemongrass (*Cymbopogon citratus/flexuosus*), Marjoram (Sweet; *Origanum marjorana*), Spanish (*Thymus mastichina*),

13

Melaleucas (Cajeput, Niaouli, Ti-tree; *Maleleuca cajuputi, M. quinque-nervia, M. alternifolia*), Melissa (*Melissa officinalis*), Moroccan Chamomile (*Ormenis mixta*), Myrrh (*Commiphora molmol*), Myrtle (*Myrtus communis*), Neroli (*Citrus aurantium flos*), Nutmeg (*Myristica fragrans*), Palmarosa (*Cymbopogon martinii*), Patchouli (*Pogostemon cablin*), Peppermint (*Mentha x piperita*), Pine (*Pinus sylvestris*), Rose (*Rosa damascena/centifolia*), Rosemary chemotypes (*Rosmarinus officinalis/Salvia rosmarinus*), Rosewood (*Dalbergia maritima*), Sandalwood (*Santalum album/spicatum*), Spruce (*Picea mariana*), Thyme chemotypes (*Thymus* sp.), Vetivert (*Vetiveria zinazoides*), Violet leaf (*Viola odorata*), Yarrow (*Achillea millefolium*), Ylang Ylang (*Cananga odorata*).

## Essential oils to be used with caution

- Basil, Exotic (*Ocimum basilicum*): May be toxic and abortifacient
- Bay Laurel (*Laurus nobilis*): Some reports of toxicity
- Bay, West Indian (*Pimenta racemosa*): Possible skin irritation and cumulative toxicity
- Bergamot (*Citrus aurantium* ssp. *bergamia*): Photosensitisation
- Black Pepper (*Piper nigrum*): Skin irritant
- Cedarwood, Atlas (*Cedrus atlantica*): Chronic toxicity
- Cinnamon leaf (*Cinnamomum zeylanicum*): Chronic toxicity, skin irritation
- Citronella (*Cymbopogon nardus*): Skin irritant
- Eucalyptus, Blue Gum (*Eucalyptus globulus*): Chronic toxicity
- Fennel, Sweet (*Foeniculum vulgaris*): Chronic toxicity
- Ginger (*Zingiber officinalis*): Skin irritant
- Hyssop (*Hyssopus officinalis*): Chronic toxicity, pinocarvone may cause fits in susceptible individuals
- Lemon (*Citrus limomum*): Skin irritation
- Lemongrass (*Cymbopogon citratus*): Skin irritant
- Lemon verbena (*Lippia citriodora*): Skin irritation in high doses (true Lemon Verbena is very hard to obtain and high in price, check the botanical name and country of origin)
- Melissa (*Melissa officinalis*): Skin irritation at high doses (also very expensive and difficult to obtain in the unadulterated form)
- Orange, Bitter (*Citrus aurantium*): Chronic toxicity, skin irritation. Sweet orange does not irritate the skin and has similar therapeutic properties, especially on the emotional level.

- Nutmeg (*Myristica fragrans*): Chronic toxicity, skin irritation
- Peppermint (*Mentha x piperita*): Skin irritation
- Thyme, phenol chemotypes (*Thymus vulgaris*): CT thymol, carvacrol

## Essential oils used exceptionally and with due caution

All these oils have toxicity issues due to various constituents such as thujone, methyl salicylate, and so forth. Although the herbs may be used safely, the oils are not recommended to be used in general.

- Ajowan (*Trachyspermum ammi*)
- Bitter Almond (*Prunus amygdalus*)
- Arnica (*Arnica montana*)
- Birch (*Betula* spp.)
- Boldo (*Peumus boldus*)
- Buchu (*Agathosma betulina*)
- Calamus (*Acorus calamus*)
- Camphor (*Cinnamonum camphora*)
- Horseradish (*Amoracia rusticana*)
- Jaborandi (*Pilocarpus microphyllus, P. jaborandi*)
- Marigold (*Tagetes* spp.)
- Mugwort (*Artemisia vulgaris*)
- Mustard (*Sinapsis alba, Brassica nigra*)
- Pennyroyal (*Mentha pulegium*)
- Rue (*Ruta graveolens*)
- Sage (*Salvia officinalis*)
- Santolina (*Santolina chamaecyparissus*)
- Sassafras (*Sassafras albidum*)
- Savin (*Juniperus sabina*)
- Tonka bean (*Dipteryx odorata*)
- White Cedar (*Thuja occidentalis*)
- Wintergreen (*Gaultheria procumbens*)
- Wormwood (*Artemisia absinthium*)

## Contraindicated essential oils

For certain conditions, the use of particular essential oils is contraindicated.

## Epilepsy

Camphor, Fennel, Hyssop, Rosemary, Sage, Wormwood.

## High blood pressure

Thyme, Rosemary, Hyssop, and Sage.

## Low blood pressure

Lavender, Ylang Ylang, and Clary Sage (unless mixed with a hypertensive oil, see above).

## Essential oil use in pregnancy

In pregnancy **avoid** Basil, Birch, Cedarwood, Clary Sage, Clove, Cinnamon, Cypress, Geranium, Fennel, Jasmine, Juniper, Sweet Marjoram, Myrrh, Nutmeg, Peppermint, Rose, Rosemary, Sage, and Thyme. Also, do not use Lavender or Chamomiles in the first trimester. When working with a woman who is breast feeding or with small infants it is also necessary to exercise caution.

The oils that are generally accepted to be quite **safe**, at reduced rates and taking into account normal precautions, during pregnancy and for small children are: Citrus (Grapefruit, Lemon, Lime, Mandarin, Orange, Tangerine), Eucalyptus, Frankincense, Ginger, Tea tree, Myrtle, Neroli, Patchouli, Petitgrains, Rosewood, Sandalwood.

Some oils are thought to antidote homeopathic remedies, and others may alter blood sugar levels.

# CHAPTER 4

# Therapeutic applications and doses

## Dosages and dilutions

With the application methods below, the dose rate is determined by the number of drops and the frequency of application. The number of drops is dependent upon the strength of the individual—i.e. less for a child, old person, or otherwise frail individual, as well as their body weight.

The frequency of application is determined by the severity of the affliction; more often at the onset, gradually reducing down with improvement.

## Methods of delivery of essential oils

### Transdermal

As you will be aware, this method of delivery is even used for some pharmaceutical preparations. The skin is the largest organ in the body, with a surface of approximately 1.8 m², which is a vast area of application. The skin is involved in respiration, absorption, and elimination. Elimination and respiration are active processes, however, absorption occurs by simple diffusion. When the skin is actively involved in elimination (e.g. in a sauna) some aromatherapists feel it is inappropriate to use essential oils, as they will not absorb adequately via the skin (however, they will still have emotional effects due to the stimulation of the olfactory system).

The outer keratinised layer, or stratum corneum (horny layer), is partly lipophilic and partly hydrophilic, meaning that it is partially permeable to both water and fat soluble molecules. Since essential oils contain small molecular weight molecules of both types, they tend to permeate the skin quite readily. Molecules over 500 molecular weight hardly penetrate at all, but since all essential oil constituents are well below this they have no problem. It would also appear that highly negative molecules increase the permeability of the skin, so essential oils with these components may be used as excipients.

What factors affect absorption into the blood stream?

- **Surface area of application**—Obviously, the larger the area of application, the more essential oil is absorbed. However, if areas are left uncovered then most of the essential oil will evaporate, rather than passing through the skin.
- **Different bodily region skin permeability**—Most permeable regions are the soles of the feet, the palms of the hands, the forehead, armpits, damaged, abraded or inflamed skin, mucous membranes, and the scalp. The least permeable areas are the buttocks, abdomen, trunk, and legs. The outer dead layers of skin cells act as a reservoir of essential oils. This means that the client should remain clothed, and avoid washing, showering etc. for about 4–5 hours after a treatment.
- **Carrier oil viscosity**—The more viscous oils such as almond and olive oil permeate more slowly, whereas a low viscosity oil, such as linseed, permeates more quickly. The fatty acid composition of the carrier oil will also affect the rate of absorption. Since most essential oils are of low viscosity they will not have an effect on the rate of absorption.
- **Hydration**—Skin that has been immersed in hot water will have enhanced absorption of certain oils (explaining the value of adding essential oils to the bath). Although the stratum corneum on the soles and the palms is many times thicker than on other parts of the body, it has a tendency to take up water. So the traditional foot bath is an

excellent system of delivery. If the skin has been previously washed with detergents it will be even more permeable.

- **Temperature**—The temperature of the oil, the skin, and the environment will all affect the rate of absorption. A rise in the temperature of the oil (by placing in a warm water bath), or skin (by bathing in warm water, applying a hot water bottle or warming with a hair drier) is sufficient to increase absorption several fold (Kielhorn, Melching-Kollmuß, Mangelsdorf, 2006) and the circulatory stimulating effect of massage will not doubt enhance this. However, massage also encourages evaporation of essential oils, thus reducing dosage.
- **Occlusion**—Covering the skin with non-permeable material will also have an effect. This does not mean that you should wrap up in cling film. Merely covering areas where application has taken place with towels and dressing in normal outdoor clothes after a treatment should suffice.
- **Ionic solutions**—Negatively charged molecules penetrate the skin more easily. This means that their inclusion in a blend can speed up the absorption process.
- Greasy ointments, especially those containing lanolin or mineral oils, will hinder the absorption of essential oils and are not suitable media for their application due to the large size of the fat molecules they contain. However, vegetable oil based lotions and creams increase the permeability of the skin by enhancing the skin's hydration and therefore are useful media, especially for the patient to use between treatments.

## Massage

Dilute in a carrier at 0–5%, depending on the individual and the condition being treated. If massage is only over a small area (for instance colonic massage for constipation), higher dosages may be used. For babies and children under six, use dilutions of 1% or less and stick to the safe oils until you have adequate knowledge—refer to oil monographs. For children between six and twelve use 1–2%.

Remember that this refers to the total amount of essential oil, not to the amount of each oil individually. If you are making a blend for a baby, you may have to make a larger amount to get the dilution low enough.

Always use vegetable oils, since mineral oils, including baby oil, form a barrier and do not allow the oils to pass into the body.

## Baths

Either full body baths or foot, hand, or sitz baths. Add between 4 and 10 drops in total, after running the water. Remember that very hot baths may make you feel weak, so a warm bath is preferable.

With babies and young children 1–2 drops are sufficient. The essential oil should be dissolved in a dispersant to prevent concentrated essential oil getting into the eyes or mucosa. Suitable dispersants are a lotion base, dispersible oil, egg yolk, full fat milk, cream, yoghurt, or a proprietary dispersant. Also, oils may be used to prepare an aromatic salt, made up of a 2:1 ratio of sea salt to Epsom salts or using either sea salt or Epsom salts alone. **The normal carrier oils are not suitable as they make the surface of the bath slippery and unsafe.** An alternative is to use hydrosols.

With children of 6–12 use 2–5 drops.

Some oils will irritate the skin if added neat to a full body bath. These include:

Citrus oils, Black pepper, Ginger, Cinnamon, Clove, Fennel, Thyme, and Peppermint. They may be used in a foot bath with caution. Again, refer to specific monographs.

## Compresses

Hot and cold compresses are prepared by adding several drops of essential oil to a gauze or face cloth that has been soaked in water. A simpler method is to prepare a blend of the oils at an appropriate dilution (0–5%), then apply to the skin, and then apply a hot water bottle, or an ice pack, wrapped in a towel to the area. A clay poultice with essential oils mixed in may also be used.

## Talcum powders

For applications to dry or irritated dermal conditions, one has the choice of hydrosols or oils dissolved in vodka, or a lotion if appropriate. Another alternative is an aromatic talc, prepared from the relevant clay or powdered herbs/arrowroot/cornflour, to which oils are added at 1% (v:v) and applied as required. These are especially good for itchy conditions, such as some eczema and chicken pox.

*Intensive blends for topical use*

In this approach, rather than using a fixed oil one uses an appropriate essential oil as an active base. An example would be to treating shingles:

1 ml Geranium (*Pelargonium graveleons*)
1 ml (*Eucalyptus citriodora*)
8 ml Tea tree (*Meleuca alternifolia*)

## Reflex point applications

There is no reductionist way of explaining how this works, but we are always astounded with the results. The essential oils are put together in a concentrated form without any carrier oil. They are then applied to the relevant reflexes on the foot.

We have seen this improve movement range in a whiplash injury in the neck within fifteen minutes; improved movement in a knee with damaged ligaments; clearing of sinuses with much movement of phlegm and little popping noises in a serious sinus problem, and many more.

There is no need to massage the oils in; one just applies them to the relevant points and then puts on some socks to encourage the oils to sink in rather than evaporate.

## Frictions

Frictions are the application of small amount of neat essential oil blends by dripping onto the palms of the hands and then friction rubbing them over the desired area of treatment.

I came upon this technique in Nelly Grosjean's book, *Aromatherapy From Provence*, and find it very useful. Frictions can be used as tonics for general health and wellbeing or to treat specific ailments or weaknesses in the constitution.

Tonic frictions can be applied in the morning to give vitality and alertness for the day, and relaxing frictions at night can help us relax from the stresses of the day and sleep better. Frictions can also be used to aid circulation, digestion, the respiratory and other systems, or to support the health of the skin, hair, and scalp.

For a 'healthy adult' the doses are:

- Body friction: 30 drops, abdominal 10–20 drops, chest and back (for respiratory conditions or back tension) 20–30 drops.
- Painful areas can be treated by applying 4–10 drops fractioned over the painful area and a little rub over the solar plexus.

Friction doses should be reduced for children under the age of fourteen, by half for children age 6–12, by a quarter for children aged 2–6 and, do not be use on children younger than two. For children with sensitive skin and frail people, mix the friction blend with an equal or greater quantity of olive oil or almond oil.

Once you have made up your friction blend, it can either be applied by putting the drops onto your hands and then massaging in a clock-wise direction over the are to be treated, or the drops can be applied to the area and then massaged in with the hands.

A blend of 3–5 oils should be used and normal cautions should be observed.

Oils particularly safe and effective to use in frictions are:

Benzoin (*Styrax benzoin*), Carrotseed (*Daucus carota*), Chamomiles (*Matricaria recutita, Anthemis nobilis*), Cedarwood (*Cedrus atlantica*), Cistus (*Cistus ladanifer*), Cypress, (*Cypressus sempervirens*), Elemi (*Canarium luzonicum*), Eucalyptus (*Eucalyptus radiata or R. smithii*), Geranium (*Pelargonium graveolens*), Immortelle (*Helichrysum italicum*), Lavender (*Lavandula officinalis*), Lemon (*Citrus limomum*), Mandarin (*Citrus recutita*), Manuka (*Leptosperum scoparium*), Sweet marjoram (*Origanum marjoranal*), Myrrh (*Commiphora molmol*), Myrtle (*Myrtus communis*), Niaouli (*Melaleuca quinquinervia*), Orange (*Citrus aurantium*), Palmarosa (*Cymbopogon martini*), Patchouli (*Pogostemon cablin*), Petitgrain (*Citrus aurantium fol.*), Pine (*Pinus sylvestris*), Ravensara (*Ravensara aromatica*), Ravintsara (*Cinnamomum camphor*), some chemotypes of Rosemary (*Rosmarinus officinalis*), Sandalwood (*Santalum album, S. spicatum*), Spruce (*Picea mariana*), Vetivert (*Vetiveria zinazoides*), Ylang Ylang (*Cananga odorata*).

There are quite a few that need diluting for frictions, such as Aniseed (*Pimpinella anisum*), Basil (*Ocimum basilicum*), Bay (*Laurus nobilis*), Bergamot (*Citrus bergamia*), Black pepper (*Piper nigrum*), Cardamom (*Elettaria cardamomum*), Cinnamon (*Cinnamomum verum*), Citronella (*Cymbopogon nardus*), Clary Sage (*Salvia sclarea*), Clove (*Eugenia cayophyllum*), Fennel

(*Foeniculum vulgare*), Ginger (*Zingiber officinale*), Juniper (*Juniperus communis*), Lemongrass (*Cymbopogon citratus, C. nardus*), May Chang (*Litsea cubeba*), Nutmeg (*Myristica fragrans*), Oregano (*Origanum vulgare*), Peppermint (*Mentha x piperita*), Rose (*Rosa centofolia, R. damascena*), Thymes (*Thymus* spp.), Valerian (*Valeriana officinalis*).

Always err on the side of caution and patch test a blend before using.

A friction blend can be used every day for up to three weeks and then should be changed.

## Inhalation

Essential oils are inhaled during a traditional treatment, but may also be inhaled from a steam bath, from a tissue, used in a vaporiser or simply sniffed from the bottle. The mucous membrane of the nose is highly permeable, as is the lining of the lung, but the amount of essential oil entering the blood stream via this route is likely to be minuscule; this is due to the small amount of oil that actually enters the nose and reaches the membranes of the nose and lungs. However, there has been shown to be a differential effect of dose, whereby pharmacological actions can be measured from tiny amounts of oil, which aren't present at higher doses—this means that smaller doses can be more effective.

Traditionally, it is thought that the main reason that essential oils have an effect through inhalation is due to molecular absorption via the mucous membrane of the nose allowing direct stimulation of the central nervous system (CNS) to produce marked effects—this includes the limbic system, responsible for mood. Due to the proximity of the limbic system to the hypothalamus and the pituitary gland, it is possible that its stimulation can also have an indirect trickle-down effect on homeostasis and the endocrine system, but this is purely hypothetical.

Due to small quantities of oil absorbed via inhalation, this is an extremely safe method of delivery, particularly for conditions of a 'nervous' origin. Toxic effects are very unlikely, although occasionally very strong reactions are observed such as a lowering in blood pressure with the aroma of oils such as Lavender or Ylang Ylang, or relief of nausea with the aroma of Peppermint, or a feeling of wellness from the aroma of Lemon or of a more positive attitude from inhaling the aroma of Roman Chamomile. Many such effects have been observed with students and patients.

Inhalation is also a valuable way of treating both the upper and lower respiratory system.

### Steam inhalations/facial saunas

Add 1–5 drops of essential oil to a bowl of boiling water. The head is covered with a towel and deep breaths are taken for about ten minutes. Start with about thirty seconds exposure and build up. Inhalations may be done up to six times a day. Alternatively, drops can be inhaled from a tissue.

### Vaporisation/room fragrancing

The amount of oil used depends on the size of the room and what effect is required, but beware of over exposure by this route. It is possible to produce undesirable side effects, such as nausea and headaches, if an oil is used for too long or too many different oils are used in a short period of time. It is better to suggest two hours maximum usage at a time.

## Internal use

In order to prescribe oils internally, a good knowledge of dose rates and toxicity is needed, and this is definitely not a method recommended for home use, whatever the oils may be diluted in. The capsules used for oral dosage in France have a slow dissolving shell which does not break down until it reaches the small intestine. This eliminates the possibility of the essential oils causing damage to the delicate lining of the oesophagus and stomach. The essential oils are also diluted in a vegetable carrier oil. This method of delivery can be useful for infections and disorders of the digestive tract. Peppermint oil capsules are used in orthodox medicine for the treatment of irritable bowel syndrome. I have observed the inhalation of Peppermint oil to be equally effective for some people.

Oral dosing carries risks. As well as the possibility of oils causing irritation to the digestive tract, large quantities of oil are carried to the liver, which may have problems breaking them down. There is also a possibility of vomiting and nausea. Also, the essential oils may be destroyed by gut enzymes, or in the liver, and malabsorption may prevent them getting where they are needed.

As well as diluting the essential oils in a base oil, honey or tahini is sometimes used. The usual rate of dilution is a maximum of three drops total of essential oil per teaspoon (5 ml) but often a far lower dose is effective (see example below). The dose is then a teaspoon up to three times a day for a maximum of three weeks, if used continuously.

For example, a digestive honey:

250 ml jar of honey
20 drops Tarragon (*Artemisa drancunculus*)
20 drops Mandarin (*Citrus reticulata*)

## Herbal pills

In this method a mixture of powders appropriate for the condition is made or else one that acts as a carrier that affords some protection for the mucosa. The oils are then added to give a dose of 1–3 drops per pill.

Our basic pill mixture always contains three parts per ten parts of Marshmallow root (*Althaea officinalis*) powder by volume. The powder is then mixed 1:2 with honey by volume to make a thick dough.

When adding the honey, one calculates how many drops of oil. We make our pills about 2 ml in volume. So, if we have made 750 ml of dough the maximum amount of oil added would be 375 drops. However, in our experience this is far more than is needed so we would add more like 100 drops (5 ml) of essential oil. This batch size makes 380 pills, approximately.

## Vaginal applications

Treatment of the female reproductive system can be successfully achieved by applying a lotion or cream to the lower abdomen and back, using a higher dilution than normal. Pessaries can be made from cocoa butter and essential oils. Because the vagina has a very delicate lining, this method is not recommended for those without medical training. Other methods include douching, insertion of a cream or applications on a tampon (definitely not neat, as one student reported to me that an aromatherapist had recommended inserting a tampon soaked in neat Tea Tree—the mere thought makes my eyes water!). Again the delicate lining of the vagina can be severely irritated if oils are not evenly dispersed.

## Rectal application

In France suppositories are routinely used as a method of application, by doctors. Its main application is for the treatment of intestinal problems where the oils may be broken down before reaching the colon. Again, it carries risks, since the lining of the rectum is highly sensitive to irritation, and the oils are carried straight into the circulation, without metabolism in the liver occurring. This is not to be recommended either.

## Gargles/mouth washes/sprays

Note that ear, nose, and throat (ENT) infections can indicate digestive problems, so pay attention to the diet and digestive function, also. Gargles and mouthwashes may be made up by diluting oils in cider vinegar, glycerine, honey, or alcohol (vodka or brandy) at 1–5%. The oils may also be mixed into sea salt to make an aromatic salt, see below. The preparation is then dissolved in warm water and used to gargle with or to wash the mouth. Use a plant spray, or dental pulsator to spray into the throat or nose. If an infection is deep in the throat, then an aromatic salt may be diluted at the rate of 9 g/litre and sprayed into the throat. Not pleasant, but very effective!

## Using essential oils in cooking and flavouring

Essential oils are widely used as flavouring ingredients by the food industry. If oils of therapeutic quality are used, this is another way to use them for health. There are some oils that should never be ingested but many can be used this way. However, do bear in mind it takes large quantities of plant material to produce essential oils so that one drop can be the equivalent of the volatile oil contained in quite large amounts of the plant material so the flavour is much stronger than you might expect. For example, to make just 1 mg of pure rose essential oil you need 50,000 individual petals (around 1500 rose flowers), which is the equivalent of around 3.5 kg (7–8 pounds) of rose petals.

Some ideas for including oils in cooking are:

One drop of rose, neroli, peppermint, mandarin essential oil in a batch of raw chocolate.

A drop of lemon oil in a batch of cake batter (or orange or rose for example).

A drop of basil oil in a batch of tomato sauce or soup.

This is too large a topic to cover in this book. However, this will be covered in a future article on our website.

## CHAPTER 5

# The chemistry of essential oils

The chemical components of essential oils can be divided into chemical classes or functional families. Within a family or class the molecules all have the same functional group, or active area. Again, if you think of the key and lock image, the functional group is the shaft of the key, and will unlock similar locks, whilst the carbon backbone is the handle, and determines the size and weight of the molecules. This means that within a functional family the molecules all have similarities, but some of the members of the class will have slightly specialised actions. The constituents of an oil are what give it its properties and uses. An oil is not just its components, the whole is more than the sum of its parts, and we must never lose sight of the fact that we are working with natural substances—the essence of the plant, which some would call its life force or soul. However, by understanding the therapeutic action of the oil's components we can predict what it can be used for, even if it is a newly discovered oil. This is what makes chemistry exciting.

In addition to the hydrocarbon chains that form the basis of the molecules, the functional group often contains elements—such as oxygen, occasionally sulphur or nitrogen. Bonds between carbon and these molecules are weaker, which means that they have a higher polarity and are more liable to react—this is why it determines the function of the molecule. The amount of effect that the functional group has on the action of the molecule depends on the size of the hydrocarbon chain. The smaller the chain, the more influence the functional group will have.

As you study the functional classes of chemicals, it is best to start off by learning the name of the class, its main therapeutic actions, and the basic structure of the functional group. As you study each oil refer back to the chemical families and check which family each constituent belongs to. This will help you to learn the chemistry and will also help you remember the properties of each oil. Setting up a card index may help.

Most of the molecules in a particular class will have similar names, although there are always the awkward exceptions to the rule. Aldehydes normally end in -al, but both alcohols and phenols may end in -ol, and there are a few that are just completely odd.

## Terpenes

These are divided in to several groups, depending on the number of carbons they contain. They follow the formula $(C_5H_8)_n$; so, for example, $C_{10}H_{16}$ molecules are the monoterpenes, $C_{15}H_{24}$ are the sesquiterpenes, and $C_{20}H_{16}$ are the diterpenes.

### Monoterpenes

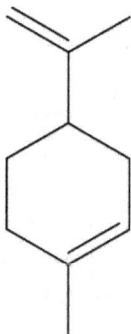

Limonene

Monoterpenes $(C_{10}H_{16})$ are the simplest molecules synthesised by plants, and therefore they occur in large numbers in more primitive plants, such as the Gymnospermae.

They are local analgesics, with a mild rubefacient action. They are antiseptic, mildly mucolytic, and expectorant. They are physically and mentally stimulating. They are adrenal cortex stimulants, which gives them a cortisone-like action (without the side effects of synthetic steroids). Correctly distilled and stored terpene-rich oils are actually soothing to the skin but irritation is caused by break down products in old or incorrectly stored terpene-rich oils, rather than the terpenes themselves. Therefore with terpene rich oils it is best to buy small amounts and use them within a year of purchase.

Camphene: Juniper, Petitgrain, Pine, Black Pepper, Nutmeg

Carene: Black Pepper

Cymene: Nutmeg (Para cymene is an aromatic terpene—it is a catalyst for bactericidal actions of other molecules, and enhances the action of terpineol in particular)

Dipentene: Bergamot, Cinnamon bud, Coriander, Fennel, Lemon, Nutmeg

Limonene: Bergamot, Fennel, Lemon, Neroli, Orange, Black Pepper Myrcene: Black Pepper

Phellandrene: Cinnamon bud, Coriander, Lemon, Peppermint, Pine, Black Pepper

Pinene: Coriander, Cypress, Eucalyptus globulus, Fennel, Pine, Rosemary, Black Pepper

Sabinene: Sweet Marjoram, Black Pepper, Nutmeg Sylvestrene: Cypress, Pine

Terpinene: Coriander, Sweet Marjoram

Thujene: Black Pepper

## Sesquiterpenes

Sesquiterpenes ($C_{15}H_{24}$) are slightly larger and more complex. As they contain a lot of double bonds, they are called polyunsaturated molecules and can help to mop up unwanted molecules, which contributes to their action. Chamazulene is one of the best known sesquiterpenes. It is a deep, dark blue colour. Sesquiterpenes are antihistamines, anti-inflammatory, and soothing and relaxing emotionally and physically. This means they are also sedative.

(Cham)azulene: German Chamomile (*Matricaria recutita*), Roman Chamomile (*Anthemis nobilis*), Wormwood (*Artemisia absinthium*), Yarrow (*Achillea millefolium*).

Cadinene: Frankincense (*Boswellia carterii*), Lemon (*Citrus limomum*), Patchouli (*Pogostemon cablin*).

Caryophyllene: Lavender (*Lavandula vera*), Sweet Marjoram (*Origanum marjorana*), Rosemary (*Rosmarinus officinalis*). Clary Sage (*Salvia sclarea*), Cinnamon Bud (*Cinnamomum verum*), Clove Bud (*Eugenia caryophyllum*).

Cedrene: Atlas Cedarwood (*Cedrus atlantica*), Juniper (*Juniperus communis*) (caryophyllene is also antiviral).

## Alcohols, phenols, acids, and aromatic aldehydes

Are all broadly termed as *hydroxylic molecules.*, meaning they contain an OH group. They are quite different structurally but are all anti-infectious and immunostimulants, as well as being very warming and stimulating. However, they vary in their strength of action and their contraindications, which gives them different applications.

### Alcohols

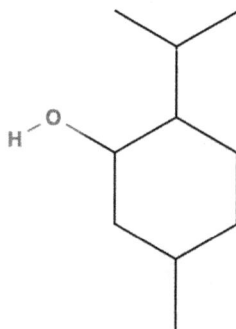

Menthol

Like the terpenes these are subdivided, according to the number of carbon atoms they contain.

### Monoterpenoid alcohols — monoterpenic alcohols/monoterpenols

One of the least toxic and non-dermocaustic groups. Their functional group is an OH group. All are pathogenic, acting against fungi, viruses, and bacteria. Their specific effectiveness will be discussed later in the course. In addition, these constituents are also diuretic and tonifying. They are also nervines. Their functional group is an oxygen and hydrogen hydroxylic group.

Borneol: Coriander (*Coriandrum sativum*), Lavender, Nutmeg (*Myristica fragrans*), Pine (*Pinus sylvestris*)

Citronellol: Geranium (*Pelargonium graveolens*), Palmarosa (*Cymbopogon martini*)

Geraniol: Palmarosa, Rose, Coriander, Geranium, Neroli, (*Citrus aurantium* flos) Nutmeg, Petitgrain (*Citrus aurantium* fol), Thyme (*Thymus vulgaris*)

Lavandulol: Lavender

Linalol: Lavender, Neroli, Nutmeg, Thyme

Menthol: (Liver stimulant, vasoconstrictor) Peppermint

Myrtenol: Geranium

Nerol: Bergamot (*Citrus bergamia*), Neroli, Petitgrain

Terpineols: Bergamot, Geranium, Sweet marjoram, Neroli

Thujanol-4: (Liver stimulant) Thyme


## Sesquiterpenoid alchohols — sesquiterpenols

These are less common than monoterpenols and are generally specific to one plant. They are not as antipathogenic, but are good immunostimulants. They are general tonics and specifically decongest the venous and lymphatic systems.

Cedrol: (Phlebotonic): Atlas Cedarwood

Farensol: Palmarosa, Rose, Ylang Ylang Nerilidol: Neroli

Patchoulol: Patchouli

Santalol (Cardiotonic): Sandalwood (*Santalum album*)

Viridiflorol (Oestrogen like, Phlebotonic): Niaouli

Carotol (Liver cell regenerator): Carrot seed


## Diterpenoid alcohols — diterpenols

These are very large molecules in comparison to other essential oil components. This means that they are not very volatile and they are only found in a few essential oils. However, they are similar in structure to human sex hormones, which makes them valuable therapeutic tools for regulating the female reproductive system. Also, note that they must be used with caution to prevent upsetting the cycle.

Sclareol: Clary Sage (*Salvia sclarea*)

Salviol: Common Sage (*Salvia officinalis*)

## Phenols

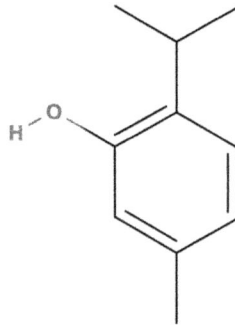

Thymol

Phenols contain a benzene ring, which makes them strong in their action and means they need to be used with some caution. They are highly effective anti-infectious tools (92% of pathogens are sensitive to phenols, including bacteria, fungi, viruses, and parasites), but that they can be dermocaustic with long-term use, and at high concentrations. Overuse can damage both mucous membranes and the liver. They should therefore be alternated with alcohols when treating chronic infections. This prevents any side effects and also means that neither the person, nor the pathogen becomes acclimatised. They are particularly useful for disinfecting the air when used in a diffuser or a burner. In common with the other hydroxylic molecules they are immuno-stimulant. They are stimulating tonics with a rubefacient action and have a reputation as sexual stimulants.

Carvacrol (most toxic): Oregano (*Origanum vulgaris*), Savory (*Satureja montana*), Thyme

Thymol: Thyme

Eugenol (may also be classified as a phenyl methyl ether; antispasmodic): Cinnamon Bud (*Cinnamomum verum*), Clove Leaf (*Eugenia caryophyllum*), Black Pepper (*Piper nigrum*), Nutmeg (*Myristica fragrans*), West Indian Bay (*Pimenta racemosa*)

## Aromatic aldehydes

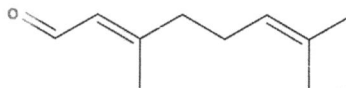

Citral

Although they have the same functional group as aldehydes, aromatic aldehydes are formed by the shikimic acid pathway and are more similar in action to phenols since they contain a benzene ring.

Anisic aldehyde: Aniseed (*Piminella anisum*), Vanilla (*Vanilla* sp.)

Cinnamic aldehyde (highly irritating to skin and mucous membranes): Cinnamon bark (*Cinnamomum verum*), Cinnamon leaf (*Cinnamomum verum*), Cassia (*Cinnamomum cassia*)

Cuminic aldehyde: Cumin (*Cuminum cyminum*)

Benzaldehyde: Benzoin (*Styrax benzoin*)

## Acids

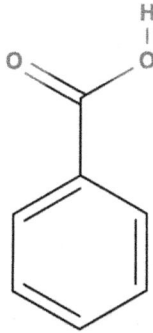

Benzoic acid

Acids are highly water soluble and are therefore present mainly in the hydrolat (hydrosol or aromatic water), giving them their own therapeutic actions, along with alcohols. Acids rarely occur in the essential oil, since they tend to react with alcohols to form esters. Most acids are non-toxic. They are excellent anti-inflammatory agents, which is why hydrolats can be so useful for skin care. They are also febrifuges and are antihypertensive. They are also calming on an emotional level.

Benzoic acid: Benzoin, Ylang Ylang (*Cananga odorata*)

Cinnamic acid: Benzoin (*Styrax benzoin*)

Citronellic acid: Citronella (*Cymbopogon nardus*), Melissa (*Melissa officinalis*)

Geranic acid: Geranium (*Pelargonium* sp.), Rose (*Rosa damescena/centofolia*)

Phenylacetic acid: Neroli (*Citrus aurantium* flos)

Valerianic acid: Valerian (*Valeriana officinalis*)

## Aldehydes

Aldehydes are excellent anti-inflammatory agents, a factor which is sometimes ignored due to the fact they are also dermal irritants at high concentrations. They are mild anti-infectious agents, particularly against bacteria and fungi, including Candida, and immuno-stimulant. They are considered to be cooling and calming to the emotions and physiological stimulants. They are febrifuges and antihypertensive. Aldehydes are also litholytic, vasodilatory, and analgesic.

Citronellal Citronella, Eucalyptus citriodora, Lemon, Lemongrass, Melissa Citrals (Neral and Geranial) also anti-viral: Melissa, Lemongrass, Geranium, Orange, Mandarin.

## Ketones

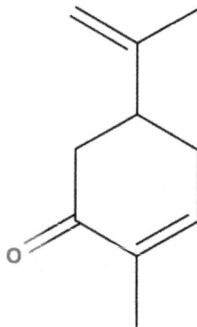

Carvone

Some ketones are highly toxic and, therefore, need to be treated with caution, particularly thujone, pulegone, and pinocamphone. When used in small doses for short periods of time ketones are cooling, calming, and sedating. However, large or repeated doses may be neurotoxic so treat with caution. On the positive side, ketones are cicatrising and dermatophilic. They are also mildly antiseptic and good immuno-stimulant. They are both lipolytic and mucolytic.

Camphor/Borneone: Camphor (*Cinnamomum camphora*), Mugwort (*Artemisia vulgaris*), Spike Lavender (*Lavandula spicata*), Cinnamon, Rosemary

Carvone (cholagogue, choloretic): Caraway (*Carum carvi*), Spearmint (*Mentha spicata*), Dill (*Anthum graveolens*) Peppermint (*Mentha x piperita*)

Fenchone: Fennel (*Foeniculum vulgare*)

Jasmone: Jasmine (*Jaminum grandiflorun*)

Menthone (Cholagogue, choloretic): Peppermint, Pennyroyal (*Mentha* pulegium) Pinocamphone (Epileptogenic): Hyssop (*Hyssopus officinalis*)

Pulegone (abortifacient); Pennyroyal, Peppermint

Piperitone: *Eucalyptus dives*

Cryptone: *Eucalyptus polybractea*

Thujone (abortifacient, neurotoxic): Mugwort, Sage, Tansy (*Tanacetum vulgare*), Thuja (*Thuja occidentalis*)

Verbenone: Rosemary, Frankincense

A group of ketones found in Immortelle (*Helichrysum italicum*) are non-toxic and highly effective against bruising.

## Esters (ethanoates)

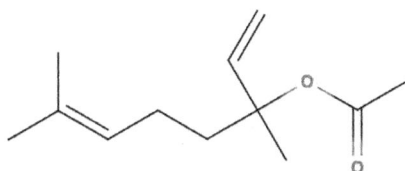

Linalyl acetate

Esters are formed by the interaction of acids and alcohols. With the exception of methyl salicylate, esters are non-toxic and non-irritant. They are also extremely calming and sedative, which makes them valuable tools for the treatment of stress related conditions, including eczema, psoriasis, insomnia, and mood swings. They are also anti-inflammatory and anti-spasmodic. They are anthelmintic and fungicidal, particularly against *Candida albicans*. They have a slight mucolytic effect. They also regulate the CNS and have an immediate effect on this system and are useful in the treatment of shock. Their names normally have two parts, the first ending in -*yl* and the second in -*ate*.

Benzyl benzoate: Benzoin, Ylang Ylang

Propyl angelate: Roman Chamomile

Geranyl acetate: Ylang Ylang

Lavandulyl acetate: Lavender

Linalyl acetate: Neroli, Lavender, Bergamot, Clary Sage, Jasmine, Lime (*Citrus* spp.)

Methyl acetate: Mandarin (*Citrus recutita*), Neroli, Orange
Octyl acetate: Frankincense
Methyl anthranilate: Mandarin, Ylang Ylang, Neroli
Methyl salicylate: Birch (*Betula* species), Wintergreen (*Gaultheria decumbens*)
Neryl acetate: Neroli
N.B. Methyl salicylate is toxic and and irritant—symptoms can include; vomiting, fever, rapid breathing, tachycardia, cyanosis, dermatitis and skin necrosis, kidney damage, internal haemorrhage due to anticoagulant potentiation of warfarin, and death.

## Phenyl methyl ethers

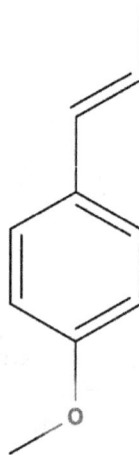

Anethole

Phenyl methyl ethers have an oestrogen-like action, which means they should be treated with the same caution as diterpenols. They are also carminative and antispasmodic. They are CNS stimulants (and also anti-depressant), which again means they need to be used with caution, as too high a dose or repeated doses can lead to overstimulation. They are rubefacient and circulatory tonics.

Anethol (trans-p-anol): Fennel, Aniseed, Star Anise (*Illicium verum*)

Estragole (Chavicol methyl ether, Methyl carvacrol) (Controversy as to the toxicity of this component): Basil (*Ocimum basilicum*), Tarragon (*Artemisia dracunculus*)

Carvacrol methyl ether: Oregano
Eugenol methyl ether: Cinamon and Clove

## Oxides

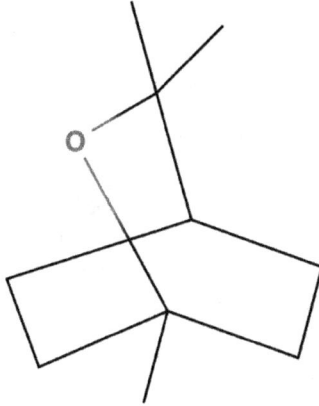

1,8-Cineole

The best expectorants. Some are also anti-infectious and effective against certain parasites. 1,8-cineole is the most commonly found and aids expiration, which can be helpful in some forms of asthma.

Bisabolol oxide: German Chamomile

Bisabolone oxide: German Chamomile

1,8-Cineole (Eucalyptole): Eucalyptus globulus, E. *polybractea, dives, radiata*, Roman Chamomile, Sweet Fennel, Lavender, Tea Tree, Nutmeg, Spanish Marjoram (*Thymus mastichina*)

## Coumarins

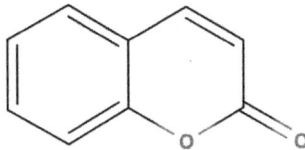

Coumarin

These molecules are fairly large and have a low volatility, and are therefore only present in oils that are distilled for a sufficient length of time or in expressed oils. They are often missing from oils prepared for the perfumery market. They are excellent sedatives, antispasmodic, anti-convulsive, antihypertensive, and also anticoagulant.

## Furanocoumarins

Bergaptene, bergamotine, and angelicine are photosensitising, which means that they sensitise the skin to UV radiation, causing increased tanning and possible burning. This occurs fifteen minutes after the application of such oils, as they take this long to reach the dermis. It is therefore advisable to avoid using these oils before exposure to UV radiation, in the form of sunbed or sunlight. It is advisable to leave a gap of 3–6 hours before exposure to UV light following application.

Angelicine: Angelica (*Angelica archangelica*)
Bergamotine: Bergamot, Lemon
Citroptene: Citrus oils
Coumarin: Lavender
Heriarin: Helichrysum, Tarragon
Ombelliferone: traces in Caraway, Coriander, Sweet Fennel

## Lactones

Lactones are large cyclic esters, which may also cause photosensitisation or skin irritation. They are strongly mucolytic and immune stimulants.

Alantolactone: Cedarwood Atlas
Bergaptene: Sweet Fennel (traces), Bergamot, Orange Petitgrain, Lemon

# CHAPTER 6

# Olfaction—the sense of smell

Olfaction and the influence of our sense of smell on our physiological and psychological responses is a study which in itself could take up several books (indeed it has) and therefore we have to limit ourselves to the salient points. I have actively endeavoured to include extensive information here on olfaction, because we tend to not to be very well connected to this sense and it is one I am particularly excited by; many people in the Western world give it little thought or try to fool it by covering up odours. This chapter includes some small vignettes and will hopefully encourage you to explore this area more to foster your understanding of the importance of this sense in the use of essential oils and in herbal medicine in general.

We smell through the left and right nostrils separately. Unlike any other nerves in the body, those involved with smell are directly connected to the same side of the brain as the stimulus and there are no synaptic junctions between the nerves and the brain. When aroma molecules are present in the air, we do not always perceive them to be affected by them; molecules present in parts per billion affect us, whereas they have to be present at parts per million in order for us to perceive them consciously. (Scheider, Singer and Singer 2018).

There are so many interesting facts about olfaction! We do not have to be familiar with a smell in order for it to elicit an emotional, mental, or physical response. Also, olfaction is a precognitive event to language; a metanym is a nonverbal communication, whilst metaphors are linguistic and a metanymic association occurs in a baby recognizing their mother's breast milk long before they can make metaphorical connections.

Although there has been intensive study of human perception of smell conducted by the perfumery industry, who have set up various study centres, smell is probably the least researched of the senses. However, research carried out into the psychology of fragrance produces some interesting results. For instance, even people who are anosmic (have no sense of smell) respond to odour; in these people physical responses and mood changes can both be measured after being exposed to various odours (Van Toller, 1999).

In Japan they found that the odour of lemons increases digestive secretions (acting on the liver, hence its reputation as a hepatic), but also makes people feel healthier and gives them a sense of wellbeing. They found introducing low levels of lemon oil into the air conditioning of some companies in Japan and America (below the level where it is consciously perceived) increased productivity by 30% (Van Toller, 1999).

Unfortunately, there is little vocabulary to express what we smell and, unlike the senses of sight and hearing, we are not encouraged to develop our appreciation (we have art and music classes at school, but no lessons in aroma!). People's perception of smell varies as much as their perception of sound and visual stimuli, thus what one person appreciates may not appeal to another. This is partially cultural. A young child is not revolted by the smell of faeces, but learns that this is 'bad'. However, in regions where wealth is measured by the number of cattle owned and cow dung is used as a building material and fuel, the smell of cow dung is thought to be pleasant. The most widely appreciated odours, however, are the floral odours.

People can also have 'blind spots' in their sense of smell, these are known as specific anosmias, where people are unable to detect certain aromas. There are also some unfortunate individuals that perceive all odours as fetid and unpleasant. This has a strong influence on their appetite. People who lose their sense of smell often find that they lose their appetite because aroma is a strong stimulus to eat (think of what happens to your appetite when you have a cold and temporarily lose the sense of smell). Digesting cooked food is quicker and gives more energy, therefore there is an evolutionary advantage to finding the smell of cooked food attractive. These aromas are called pyrazines or roasting notes, and this is why they barbeque chickens and bake bread in supermarkets, in order to make us feel hungry and buy more. People with no sense of smell also often experience depression, since smell is closely tied to the part of our brain that governs emotional responses.

It is possible to educate one's nose to be able to pick up a wider range of aromas. The easiest aromas from essential oils to decipher are those of the citrus family (they are monoterpene based and therefore are small simple molecules). However, perfumiers spend many years training their noses and building up a bank of fragrance memories, which enable them to create blends on paper. The majority of perfumiers are men. This not because they have a more acute sense of smell—women's sense of smell tends to be more acute (Brand and Millot, 2001; Dalton et al., 2002; Herz and Inzlicht, 2002). However, in women the sense of smell is influenced by their hormone levels (think of how during pregnancy women often react far more strongly to odours), and therefore varies with their cycle. One study showed that if women are using the contraceptive pill when they meet their partner then stop taking it in order to conceive, they may no longer find his smell appealing (not consciously though) and therefore split up with him (van Toller, *pers. comm.*). There are many more interesting vignettes about how the lives of highly civilised people are affected by this neglected sense and its 'primitive' influences.

When we inhale any substance two things happen—some of the molecules travel with the inhaled air to the lungs and travel across the epithelial layer of the alveoli and thence into the blood stream along with the inhaled oxygen, if they are small enough. Even if they are not, there are also taste receptors in the lungs (and many other tissues), so we actually taste the air with our lungs too (Kinnamon, 2011). However, a second process occurs, that of smelling.

The nose is the organ of olfaction and the olfactory cells are positioned at the top of the nose. This is why the deep sniff is the preferred method of getting a true odour. When the air enters the nose, it is warmed and filtered by the nasal hairs and some molecules are dissolved in the mucus; in order for this to happen they must have a molecular weight of 15–397, be volatile, chemically reactive, and soluble in water or lipids. Once dissolved they come into contact with the olfactory cells, which waft around in the mucus. The cells are either stimulated by the vibrational energy of the molecules or by their shape (or probably a combination of the two) and send a message to the brain. The cells are unusual in that there are no synapses between them and the limbic area of the brain. There are differently shaped cells that can differentiate between different aromas. Each olfactory receptor cell has a life cycle of about twenty-eight days. Sensitivity of smell generally decreases with age, due to the fact that their turnover becomes slower.

As there are no synapses between the nose and the brain, the message is passed directly and quickly via the olfactory bulb. It is received by the limbic system, which is a very ancient part of the brain. It is often described as primitive since it is involved in basic responses, such as the emotions, appetite, intuition, and memory. However, according to Richard Cytowic (2003) it is the co-evolution of the limbic system and the cerebrum which gives humans their powers of reasoning and morality. Our reasoning and logic are not solely based in the cerebrum, but are a result of an interaction between the two regions, involving more intuitive input than previously thought. This opens up all sorts of ideas about how our behaviour and reasoning are affected by aromas. It also makes clear why the use of essential oils has gained so much popularity, acting as they do on both a physical and an emotional level. It also brings up intriguing ideas of how far reaching the 'mood enhancement' effect could be, especially given the stresses of modern life and the fact that our environments are filled with so many synthetic and polluting odours.

The olfactory bulb also connects closely with the hypothalamus, which is the part of the brain considered to govern homeostasis and the endocrine system. Smell could therefore influence many of our physiological processes. There are amazing implications as to how this could initiate 'trickle down' effects on an emotional and physical level if the effects on the hypothalamic region by the olfactory bulb do illicit changes in our homeostatic and neuroendocrine responses.

Although the effect of aroma is immediate our perception of odour *fades* quickly or sensitises. This is why we cannot smell a perfume after wearing it for a while or are not aware of the aroma of cooking in the kitchen after a few minutes unless we leave the room and re-enter. It only takes forty-two molecules entering the nose and stimulating the ciliae for us to notice an aroma. We normally notice an aroma if there are 1:million parts in the air; however, emotional responses can be elicited by 1:billion.

Our sense of smell also *tires* easily. If we smell many odours in quick succession our olfactory receptors become desensitised and our nose loses the ability to detect anything consciously; this is probably a protective mechanism to prevent us being overwhelmed by too much information, sensory gating (for some people this does not happen and they do get overwhelmed). When smelling herbs (especially when working with essential oils), it is, therefore, important to take breaks. You may also need to drink plenty of water and ensure that you keep blood sugar levels up due to the physical effects of the aromas on excretion and appetite. The molecules that stimulate the olfactory nerves in this way do not enter the brain tissue; the effect is purely a nervous response, in a similar way that the stimulation of sound or vision works.

However, when an aroma is perceived some of the molecules will pass through the respiratory system, down the trachea, into the bronchi and into the lungs. As mentioned earlier, some of these are small enough to pass through the walls of the alveoli in the process known as internal respiration. They, therefore, enter the blood stream and are carried around the body and some will cross the blood-brain barrier and enter the CNS. Only tiny amounts of some of these are necessary to have an effect on the nervous system. This means that it is possible that some of the emotional effects are due to these factors. Since all the cells of our body contain neuropeptide receptors (meaning that all neurological responses are not mediated by the brain but can be elicited more locally in the tissues), it is possible that some of the effects on the nervous system are via these pathways as well as by the direct stimulation of the olfactory nerves. However, as stated above, the olfactory sense has been much neglected by physiologists and psychologists, but one interesting fact that has been uncovered is that we need a familiar smell environment in order to feel happy (Delplanque et al., 2008).

Odour has not always been so neglected by medicine. The Greeks believed that various aromas had certain healing properties—the scent of apples was good for headache and migraine, narcissi were a strong narcotic. Doctors also used to use smell in a different way. The odour of the patient was used in diagnosis; infections, such as the plague and typhoid, give the patient a particular body odour, as does depression and schizophrenia and many other conditions. In many traditional systems of medicine, the odour of the patient is still used to help form the diagnosis. Humans produce *semiochemicals* as well as pheromones. These do not elicit a specific response; they just send out a signal (semiotic means signalling).

We perceive smell via the first cranial nerve or olfactory nerve; however, there are other structures involved:

The trigeminal nerve is involved in some smell and taste experiences. For example, with black pepper or chilli a branch of the trigeminal nerve is irritated, adding to the spiciness of the taste and smell, with menthol-containing tastes and odours, the nerve gets a cooling stimulus, which adds to the cool fresh taste and smell of peppermint. Since the trigeminal nerve extensively enervates the face, this explains how some aromas seem to affect the whole face such as a sense of the whole face warming or cooling or relaxing. There are two other structures that are involved in some species; the septal organ and the vomernasal (or Jacobson's) organ. This is what a snake or a cat is using when it opens its mouth widely, in a seeming yawn, whilst in fact smelling the air—Flaymsan's response. It is also active from about the fifth month in the womb in humans, allowing the baby to 'smell' the amniotic fluid. It was thought that it turned off at birth, however more recent work suggests it stays active in many people, giving them a rather different perception of smell. The brain is divided into the reptilian, palaeomammalian, and neomammalian regions. The olfactory system feeds into the limbic system (rhinocephalon), which lies in the paleomammalian area in the nonverbal part of the brain. This region is above the reptilian brain, but below the neomammalian region. It has fifty-four areas and thirty-three pathways. This area is also associated with eating, drinking, sleep, sexual activity, memory, and emotional response. Therefore, smell can control behaviour and moderate it. Complex behaviour can be governed by smell (without involving cognitive function, thinking about whether to respond to the smell). The limbic system is primarily unconscious with no linguistic expression. The left hemisphere is the motor area for language (linguistics, consciousness, conscious, self, defence mechanism), the right is awareness, unconscious self—in other words, the right appreciates and the left describes.

It takes us longer to name smells than colours or sounds. There are many difficulties in getting an objective evaluation of odours. All sensory perception is subjective and there are additional hiccups with odour. Firstly, we do not have a descriptive language for smell. We normally rely on descriptions from the other senses—colour, taste, tone, or comparisons; "it smells like orange, mint". Smell is also affected by age, the stage of the menstrual cycle in women, trigeminal components in an odour, and the fact that we have a nasal cycle, which means the capacity to sense smells alternates between the two nostrils during the day with one nostril getting a stronger response at a time. We find that even when we pick up an odour there are huge differences in the threshold of sensitivity—up to twenty times. Another complicating factor is that after about one minute the mechanism adapts and the threshold for perceiving a smell rises, so that the level of perception is reduced by 70% from the sensory innervation (Schneider, Singer and Singer 2018). This does not happen so markedly with sound and sight, but happens appreciably with taste and touch, probably because our environment would otherwise be intolerable. We also adapt, and masking can occur. Interestingly, with certain psychological problems, neurological disease (e.g. epilepsy), and under the influence of hallucinogens, we can have olfactory hallucinations. We do not tend to think that we have the ability to summon up a smell memory in the way that we can recall memories of our other senses, but it is possible to develop the ability—this is how it is possible for a perfumier to design a new blend on paper.

Some people are synaesthetic, possibly as many as one in twenty-three. This means that they experience a cross over between their sensory modalities so that smells may have colours or sounds and so forth. The condition may be due to dominance of the limbic system; it can lead to a certain amount of defensiveness due to difficulty in communicating in the civilised world. Synaesthesia can be induced by psychoactive substances; but some researchers posit the possibility that synaesthesia is actually our natural way of being. This is explored in some depth by Richard Cytowic (2003).

Influences of smell can be very subtle. The fact that menstrual synchrony occurs has been shown to have an olfactory basis. In the same way, if female piglets are exposed to the scent of a boar they will reach puberty prematurely, and indeed, women who work with boars find that boar 'taint' is so strong in effect that it can affect their menstruation.

Unlike colour and music, we do not have a good working model of nomenclature for smells. We tend to use words such as fruity, flowery, burnt, spicy, and resinous. We can divide odour compounds into families of similar aromas or similar chemical structures. It is likely that there are different types of olfactory receptor cells, which pick up the different odour groups and it is possible that their activity can increase and that we can learn to tune this sense.

For any aroma there is a detection threshold and a higher recognition threshold; at the lower level we know we are smelling something but there needs to be sufficient quantity of molecules present for us to recognise what we are smelling; training and practice can definitely hone the ability to identify at a lower level and definitively differentiate between similar smells. Most of the research into olfaction is subjective rather than objective; memories associated with specific smells can dictate whether they are perceived as pleasant or unpleasant; if your grandmother baked apple pie with cinnamon and also was very cruel in her behaviour to you then these smells will elicit a negative response; if she was caring and loving then they will provoke a more pleasant association.

## Olfaction and the psychology of fragrance

Every culture since the beginning of time has recognised the significance of fragrance and used perfumes for pleasure, religious purposes, and therapeutics. Culturally, perfumery has fashions and trends and the skill of the perfumier is recognised as an art.

Perfumes for pleasure have often been designed as sexual attractants. Formerly the scents used heightened the smell of our pheromones and therefore extracts from the scent glands of animals were used, such as musk, ambergris, and civet. It is said that when Josephine's (Napoleon Bonaparte's wife) boudoir was redecorated after her demise, the workmen were nauseated by the heavy aroma of musk that came from the walls. However, fashions changed and in the reign of Louis 15th floral scents become more popular. Instead of heightening the smell of pheromones, they were designed to cover them. Perfumes were used to fragrance the body, but also clothing and decor. Perfumiers made scented gloves and fabrics.

It is interesting to note that perfumes are either used to amplify erogenous odours, or to mask the anti-erotic unpleasant elements of body odour. It is in relatively recent history that deodorising and masking one's personal odours has become fashionable. Alain Corbin (1986) puts forwards various theories as to the sociological changes that led to this.

### Body odour

The odour from an individual, when clean and naked, is made up of various odours from different areas of the body. The odours from the anus and genitals are normally perceived as anti-erogenous (although this perception of the latter is relatively recent). The erogenous elements of body odour are produced from the armpits, hairy pubic area, and the head.

The odour arises from the saturated fatty acids with hydrocarbon chains of four to nine carbons in length. The axillae produce the most pungent aroma made up of acids with 4–7 carbons. The pubis produces a lighter odour, made up of 7–9 carbon fatty acids. The odour of the head is much less noticeable and less pungent.

A person's odour will be affected by their colouring, particularly the colour of their hair. Obviously, there are people with intermediate colouring and this means that their odour will be between those described for the absolute types.

The odour will also be affected by diet—if you change your diet, you may well find that your body odour changes. Environment and mode of dress can also affect odour. The latter because fabrics have a filtering effect on odour.

In a concentrated form, these odours are repugnant. However, in a dilute form they can be used to trigger pleasant associations.

## Erogenous fragrance materials

As mentioned above, the first fragrance materials that were used in Europe to amplify body odours were musk, civet, and ambergris. In their undiluted form they are nauseating, but in small amounts they become very appealing. 'White musk' is the most popular of the Body Shop fragrances and is a synthetic version of the aroma of musk. Ambergris is most similar in fragrance to head hair and brown pubic hair. Musk is sweet, with a hint of ammonia and a decidedly animal element. Civet has a sharp sweet fragrance with faecal tones.

Most people find it disturbing when they discover that faecal notes are actually pleasant to most people in small amounts. It seems to be a chemical known as indole that is the key. Indole is found in human faeces and is a large acyclic ketone. It is also found in Jasmine, Neroli, and various other floral odours. One fragrance company has recently developed a product to use in washrooms. It is a Jasmine aroma with the indole removed. The missing note is produced in the environment and this gives a fully rounded aroma, masking the indole aroma.

There are other essential oils that are reminiscent of body odours.

# CHAPTER 7

# The art and therapeutics of blending

B lending oils for therapeutic use is a skill that combines both knowledge of the molecular content or character of the essential oils and creativity, so that the blend will work well and also smell appealing. If the aroma of the blend is pleasant to the user it will reinforce the therapeutic effect of the blend by giving mood enhancement and emotional benefits, which we know from psychoneuroimmunoendocrinology.

Aromatherapy normally uses 3–5 essential oils blended to give a rounded and holistic prescription for the individual being treated. It is important to realise that normally 3–5 oils are sufficient to give the therapeutic actions for the client if chosen well, but sometimes a more complex formula is needed to address the needs of the individual, so I have sometimes used up to nine essential oils in a prescription; most of the time I use five.

Some of the principles of blending are taken from perfumery. Whilst these are valid, they are not of prime consideration. Blending successfully on a therapeutic level is not a skill that can be taught. It is developed by practice and with an in-depth knowledge of the substances being used. Therefore, get to know the oils intimately and use every opportunity to make up blends for different people and different problems.

## Considerations when blending

### Safety

Firstly, are there any contraindications for the patient, such as high blood pressure, pregnancy, or the other factors mentioned in the chapter on essential oil safety?

Secondly, remember that using two oils with the same precautions means that there is twice as much potential for that effect—e.g. a blend with Lemon (*Citrus limomum*) and Bergamot (*C. bergamia*) should only contain these at the total safe amount, since both are photosensitising.

### Time of day

Sedative oils should be used sparingly or balanced with stimulating oils for morning use and vice versa.

### Therapeutic considerations

What are the presenting conditions on all levels—physical, emotional, mental or spiritual?

Are there any long-term conditions that need to also be considered?

### Aesthetic

Aesthetic blending is producing a pleasing aroma with the blend that appeals to the person who is going to use it. Personal preferences are influenced by our culture and fashions, by formed associations and memories (which can be quite unexpected), and by an individual's genetics—there is a whole area of psychology associated with fragrance. It is beyond the scope of this book to provide and exhaustive list of considerations for aesthetic blending, so we shall concentrate on the fundamental principles.

### a) Top, Middle, and Base Notes

This concept is taken from perfumery, and lays out aromas on a scale, similar to musical notes. It was developed by a French perfumier called Pus.

Top notes are sharp, penetrating, and 'light'—e.g. citrus oils. Middle notes are softer, give a mellow aroma, and would include Chamomile, Lavender, and Sweet Marjoram.

Bass notes are deep and heavy smelling. Good examples are Sandalwood, Patchouli, and Vetivert (*Vetiveria zinazoides*).

Some oils contain all three elements, such as Clary Sage and Ylang Ylang.

Always remember than if someone finds an aroma objectionable it will not do as good a job as an alternative that they find pleasant. If you are not sure whether a blend will work, experiment with drops on cotton buds or smelling strips. Intuition plays a part too but is honed by knowing the aroma and therapeutics of the oils intimately and thoroughly. Multiple molecules with a similar effect may be used to give a broader therapeutic action—e.g. in a chronic respiratory infection it is necessary to break down mucus, fight the infection, and perhaps add a catalyst to speed action.

Therefore, in this instance I would include the following components:

- Cineole rich oils to speed up absorption, break down mucus, and expectorate
- Terpenes to energise and for deep mucolysis
- Ketones for mucolysis
- Peppermint as catalyst
- Alcohols as anti-infectious

An example recipe:

8 ml Cajeput (*Melaleuca cajeputi*)

2 ml Black spruce (*Picea mariana*)

2 ml Eucalyptus (*Eucalyptus dives*) piperitone/piperitol (neurotoxic so low dose)

1.5 ml Rosemary borneone (neurotoxic, but also liver stimulant)

1.5 ml Tea Tree (*Melaleuca alternifolia*)—a low dose is used in the absence of acute infection

5 drops Peppermint as a catalyst, but a low dose to prevent too much cooling

## Individual prescriptions

This concept comes from the work of Margeurite Maury and can be a little difficult to grasp. It approaches the formulation of a blend for a patient from a very different angle. The idea is to create a blend for the individual that will change and evolve over the course of time (so what's different, I hear you say?).

The difference is that she endeavoured to formulate the oil blend so that the person's strong areas were echoed in the blend and that there was support for the weak areas.

For example, a vivacious, exotic personality might be echoed with oils such as Jasmine or Ylang Ylang, whilst an underlying lack of confidence in their femininity might be supported with Rose or Geranium; and a tendency towards mental laziness stimulated by Lemon, Grapefruit, or Rosemary.

# CHAPTER 8

# Essential oil profiles

*Basil (Ocimum basilicum)*

**Family:** Labiatae/Lamiaceae

The European variety, normally grown in France is preferable for therapeutic use, since it has a lower methyl chavicol content than the plant produces when grown in the tropics or India. Steam distilled from the flowering herb. The best quality oil is produced in France, but also oil is produced in Italy, Egypt, Bulgaria, Hungary, and the US. Exotic Basil is the same botanically, but contains more eugenol and methyl chavicol. It is also known as Reunion basil. An oil is also distilled in India from the Holy Basil (*Ocimum sanctum*). The oil is white to pale yellow.

**Constituents:** Monoterpenes (2%); pinene, camphene, ocimene, cymene, terpine. Sesquiterpenes; isocaryophyllene, $\beta$-caryophyllene, $\beta$-elemene. Monoterpenols; linalol (40–55%), fenchyl alcohol (3–12%), terpineol-4, $\alpha$ terpineol, citronellol, geraniol, hexanol. Esters; linalyl acetate, fenchyl acetate, methyl cinnamate, terpinyl acetate. Phenols; eugenol (1–19%). Phenyl ethers; methyl-chavicol (3–31%), methyl eugenol (1–9%). Ketones; borneone (0.1%).

**Actions:** Analgesic, anthelmintic, anti-inflammatory, antiseptic, anti-spasmodic, antibacterial, antiviral, cardiotonic, carminative, digestive tonic, eupeptic, fungistatic, hypertensor, insecticidal, hepatic, nervine, nervous system regulatory, reproductive decongestant.

**Uses:** Gout, migraine, rheumatoid arthritis, threadworms, wasp stings, intestinal infections, gastritis, gastric spasm, muscle cramp, viral hepatitis, cystitis (coliform), arrhythmias, arteriosclerosis, tachycardia, flatulence, sluggish digestion, stimulates digestive secretions, ulcers, hypotension, hepatobiliary deficiency, debility, mental strain, convalescence, depression, anxiety, epilepsy, nervous insomnia, nervousness, travel sickness, vertigo, uterine and prostatic congestion, dry eczema. Not emmenagogic.

## Bay Laurel (Laurus nobilis)

**Family:** Lauraceae

An evergreen tree that grows up to twenty metres. Bay is native to the Mediterranean and cultivated in France, Spain, Italy, Morocco, Yugoslavia, China, Israel, Turkey, and Russia. Oil is mainly produced in Yugoslavia from the leaves. Extensively used as a culinary herb.

**Constituents:** Monoterpenes; $\alpha$ and $\beta$ pinene, sabinene. Sesquiterpenes; $\beta$ elemene, $\beta$-caryophyllene, $\alpha$-humulene. Monoterpene alcohols; linalol, $\alpha$-terpineol, terpine-1-ol-4, borneol, geraniol, thujanol-4. Esters; terpenyl formiate, acetate, caproate, isobutyrate and isovalerate, linalyl acetate, bornyl acetate, geranyl acetate. Phenols; eugenol, cis-eugenol. Phenyl methyl ethers (PME) eugenol methyl ether. Oxides; 1,8 cineole. Lactones; costunolide, artemorine.

**Actions:** Anti-catarrhal, expectorant, mucolytic, anti-infectious, bactericide, viricide, fungicide, antispasmodic, vasodilator, modulating nervine, analgesic, anticoagulant.

**Uses:** stomatitis, mouth ulcers, viral hepatitis, enterocolitis, flu, upper respiratory infections, tonsillitis, dyspepsia, flatulence, loss of appetite, scanty periods, arthritis, rheumatism, muscular aches and pains, muscle spasms, viral neuritis, skin infections.

**Cautions:** Avoid in pregnancy and for small children. Can cause dermatitis in some individuals. May be mildly narcotic, so use in moderation.

## West Indian Bay (Pimenta racemosa)

**Family:** Myrtaceae

Native to the West Indies, a tropical evergreen tree up to eight metres in height, has large leathery leaves, and aromatic fruit. The fruits are used as a spice (allspice), whilst the oil is distilled from the leaves.

**Constituents:** Phenols; eugenol (up to 56%), chavicol. Terpenes; myrcene, limonene. Alcohols; linalool.

**Actions:** Analgesic, anti-convulsant, antineuralgic, anti-rheumatic, antiseptic, astringent, expectorant, stimulant.

**Uses:** As a scalp stimulant to prevent thinning of the hair and promote healthy hair growth, also for dandruff and greasy or lifeless hair. Arthritis, muscular and joint aches and pains, neuralgia, poor circulation, rheumatism, sprains, strains, colds, flu, and infectious diseases.

**Cautions:** Avoid in pregnancy and small children, due to high phenol content. Also, the general precautions with phenol rich oils. May be hypertensive.

## Benzoin (Styrax benzoin)

**Family:** Styracaceae

From the same plant as the widely known Friar's Balsam, used for inhalations. The gum is also known as gum Benjamin. It is exuded from the tree as a wound response to heal the tree, in common with the resins from Frankincense and Myrrh. It is therefore interesting to note that these three resins are used to heal wounds, both of the skin and the psyche.

**Constituents:** Aldehyde, aromatic; vanillin. Acids (10–20%); benzoic acid, cinnamic acid. Esters; benzyl cinnamate.

**Actions:** Anti-inflammatory, antiseptic, carminative, deodorant, diuretic, expectorant, sedative, vulnerary.

**Uses:** Its primary action is that of healing both the skin and the psyche. It is used for sore, chapped, irritated, and dry skin conditions. It's soothing and warming actions also make it useful for asthma, coughs, bronchitis, laryngitis, and urinary infections.

It is a gently cleansing oil that can help to clear wind, mucus and urine from the system. This makes it a remedy for flatulence, indigestion, and 'toxic' conditions, such as gout, arthritis, and rheumatism.

Emotionally it is warming and comforting. It is excellent for anxiety (it's sweet smell particularly appeals to children), and for grief and loneliness. It blends very well with rose for this purpose. Corresponds to the base chakra. It was traditionally used to drive out devils.

**Cautions:** Occasional reports of sensitisation in some individuals already allergic to other products. This may be due to using a resin that has been diluted in an irritating solvent. Benzoin is solid at room temperature and is therefore sold dissolved in an appropriate solvent. Although in Europe benzyl benzoate or wood alcohol are usually used, oil prepared in other countries may use low grade wood alcohol or benzene-related compounds.

### Bergamot (Citrus bergamia per./Citrus aurantium var. bergamia)

**Family:** Rutaceae

The oil is expressed from the rind of a small green fruit, similar to an orange. There are many companies that offer a furanocoumarin free (FCF) oil, which has had the bergaptene removed. Whilst this prevents phototoxicity, it is not a whole oil and has been subjected to rectification, making it unsuitable for use in true aromatherapy. The oil is used to flavour Earl Grey tea.

**Constituents:** Monoterpenes; pinenes, camphene, limonene, sabinene, myrcene, carene, cymene, and terpinene. Sesquiterpenes; bisabolene. Alcohols: linalol, nerol, geraniol, terpineol. Esters; linalyl acetate, geranyl acetate, neryl acetate. Aldehydes; geranial, neral. Coumarins; bergamotine, bergaptene.

**Actions:** Analgesic, antidepressant, anti-infectious, antiseptic, antispasmodic, aperitif, antiviral, antibacterial, calming, cicatrisant, deodorant, disinfectant, mild expectorant, febrifuge, insecticide, nervine, sedative, stomachic, tonic, photosensitiser.

**Uses:** Abscess, acne, bronchitis, carbuncle, colic, cystitis, depression, diphtheria, eczema, fevers, flatulence, gallstones, glossitis, gonorrhoea, halitosis, herpes, leucorrhoea, nervous tension, psoriasis, respiratory tract, infections, scabies, skincare, stomatitis, tonsilitis, urinary tract infections, vaginal pruritis, varicose ulcers, wounds, ulcers.

The main area of use for bergamot are as an antiseptic, in skin care and as an antidepressant. It has an antiviral action against *Herpes simplex* virus, making it valuable in the treatment of cold sores and herpes. It is also effective to treat shingles and chicken pox. One of the best preparations is to dissolve the oil in vodka or Calendula tincture and paint it onto the affected area. The evaporation of the alcohol has a cooling, analgesic effect. Its antiseptic action can be helpful in chest infections, where it's expectorant action also comes into play. It also is effective for cystitis and urethritis, as it is effective against staphylococcal and streptococcal infections. As an antidepressant, Bergamot oil can be helpful with loss of appetite associated with nervous upset and has been used to help people trying to overcome anorexia nervosa. Bergamot may alleviate premenstrual mood swings and exam nerves. Its aroma is uplifting yet calming. This, combined with its action on the digestive system makes it a valuable oil for all gastric problems associated with spasm and tension. In skin care, Bergamot oil is useful for the treatment of oily skin and acne, where it's antidepressant qualities can also be helpful to the insecure teenager. It is also healing to the skin and can be used to help heal scars, including those left by acne. Price (1991) cites it's photosensitising action as being useful in the treatment of vitiligo. A more usual application would be in the treatment of psoriasis, although this is a notably intractable condition, the treatment of which requires much patience on behalf of the patient and the therapist. It may also be useful in treating gum disorders and sore throats.

**Cautions:** Bergamot oil photosensitises the skin—therefore, it should not be used in the twelve hours preceding exposure to sunlight, sunbeds, or other UV light.

## Black Birch (Betula lenta/Betula capinefolia)

Also known as Sweet birch, Birch bark, American Black, or Cherry Birch. Steam distilled from the tree bark and mainly produced in Canada. Should be carefully sourced since there is widespread adulteration with synthetic methyl salicylate. The oil does not actually occur in the living tissue of the tree but is produced by decomposition in warm water.

**Constituents:** Esters (98%); methyl salicylate (often adulterated with synthetic methyl salicylate as is Wintergreen, which is nearly impossible to source as the natural oil).

**Actions:** Analgesic, anticoagulant, anti-inflammatory, antipyretic, antiseptic, antirheumatic, astringent, depurative, disinfectant, diuretic, diaphoretic, febrifuge, hepatic, insecticide, rubefacient, vulnerary.

Valerie Worwood (1990) recommends it for gout, rheumatism, eczema, ulcers. Julie Lawless (1992) suggests using it for skin; dermatitis, dull or congested skin, eczema, hair care, psoriasis.

For circulation, muscles, joints; toxins, arthritis, cellulite, muscle pain, obesity, oedema, poor circulation, rheumatism.

**Uses:** Recommended for muscular aches and pains, arthritis, rheumatism, and tendonitis, including tennis elbow. Davis (1988) also uses it for cellulite and oedema.

Black Birch has been suggested for various skin conditions, such as congested skin, acne, rashes, ulcers, cellulite. However, it is not suitable to be used on sensitive or damaged skin.

Since it aids the elimination of uric acid it could be used for gout, sore muscles as a counter-irritant, arthritis, epicondylitis, cramps, and lumbago.

**Caution:** Although methyl salicylate is an ester, and these are generally thought of as gentle and safe components, this one is an exception! Methyl salicylate is also the main component of Wintergreen oil, which is not used by the majority of aromatherapists due to its toxicity. Methyl salicylate has an anticoagulant action and, therefore, must never be used on patients taking Warfarin or other blood thinning medicines, since it may cause a tendency for haemorrhage. It is similar in action to salicylic acid, which is what aspirin is. The oil can also irritate the skin due to its intense warming action and should not be used on infants or during pregnancy and lactation. Should always be used at low concentrations. It is rapidly absorbed by the skin and so can even be toxic by this route.

## Black Pepper (Piper nigrum)

**Family:** Piperaceae

Steam distilled from the dried and crushed peppercorns. The oil has a pale green tinge. Occasionally light and heavy oils are offered. These are incomplete distillations and, therefore, not for aromatherapeutic use. Some companies offer a Green Pepper oil, distilled from the unripened and undried fruit—it is therapeutically similar. Mainly produced in India, Indonesia, Malaysia, China, and Madagascar. The oil is also distilled in Europe and USA from dried corns.

**Constituents:** Monoterpenes; pinene, thujene, sabinene, terpinene, carene, myrcene, limonene, phellandrene, elemene, cymene, terpinene, terpinolene, camphene. Sesquiterpenes; β-caryophyllene, humulene, guaiene, cubene, selinenes, bisabolene, calamenen, copaene, farnesene, zingiberene, bergamotene, curcumene. Monoterpenols terpineol-4, $\alpha$-terpineol, linalol, trans pinocarveol, elemol, bisabolol. Phenyl ethers; cymene methyl ether, carvacrol methyl ether, myristicin, trace, safrole trace. Ketones; carvone trace, piperitone trace. Aldehydes; piperonal. Oxides; caryophyllene oxide.

**Actions:** Analgesic, anticatarrhal, antiseptic, antispasmodic, anti-toxic, carminative, digestive, diuretic, eupeptic, expectorant, febrifuge, laxative, rubefacient, splenetic, stimulant, stomachic, tonic, especially beneficial for the spleen.

**Uses:** Eupeptic action makes it helpful for diarrhoea, loss of appe-tite, nausea, and vomiting. Black pepper's action on the liver also assists. Helps to loosen catarrh, and, therefore, used for colds, coughs, flu, chronic bronchitis, laryngitis, fevers. Before exercise, Black Pepper oil can be included in a rub to warm muscles and improve tone. After exercise, it can help relieve muscle pain. Also, use for rheumatism and toothache. The splenetic action makes it indicative for after heavy blood loss or severe bruising or with anaemia to stimulate new blood cell pro-duction. Good for lifting blends. It is a urinary antiseptic but should be avoided where the kidneys are inflamed. Seems to stimulate the pan-creas as well. Use for; catarrh, cholera, cold, colic, constipation, cough, diarrhoea, dysentery, dyspepsia, dysuria, fever, flatulence, heartburn, flu, loss of appetite, nausea, quinsy, toothache, vertigo, vomiting. For circulation, muscle, joints; anaemia, arthritis, aches and pains, neuralgia, poor circulation and muscle tone, rheumatic pain, sprains, and stiffness. Respiratory; catarrh and chills. Digestive; colic, constipation, diarrhoea, flatulence, heartburn, loss of appetitie, and nausea. Immune; colds, flu, infections, and viruses. Davis (1991) uses it for clearing energy blocks and for helping people to move on when they feel stuck. It can help to promote alertness and concentration.

**Cautions:** Care should be taken in pregnancy, skin sensitisation, kidney disease.


## Blue Cypress (Callitris intratropica)

**Family:** Cupressaceae

A medium to large tree (15–45 m) with highly fragrant wood, found in Northern Australia. The main part used to distil oil is the wood, although the bark can also yield an oil.

**Constituents:** Guaiazulene, guaiol (20–30%), guaienes, selinenes, eudedesmols, β-elemene, furanones.

**Actions:** Antibacterial, anti-inflammatory, vulnerary, analgesic, anti-irritant, and antiviral.

**Uses:** Allergic hives, insect bites, rheumatoid arthritis, general joint pain and swelling, nappy rash, erythema, common warts and verrucae, shingles, cold sores, and burns.

## Cajeput (Melaleuca leucandendron/cajeputi)

**Family:** Myrtaceae

The oil is extracted by steam distillation from the fresh leaves and twigs. The oil may have a light green colour due to traces of copper. Mainly produced in the Far East and Malaysia.

**Constituents:** Monoterpenes; pinenes, limonene. Sesquiterpenes; β-caryophyllene. Monoterpenols; viridiflorol, nerolidol. Phenols; eugenol. Oxides; 1,8-cineole (main constituent).

**Actions:** Analgesic, antimicrobial, antispasmodic, antiseptic, anthelmintic, diaphoretic, carminative, expectorant, insecticide, sudorific, and tonic.

**Uses:** In common with the other melaleucas, Cajeput is used for colds, flus, and other viral infections. It can also be used for skin infections, including acne and spots, and can be helpful for oily skin. As an anti-infectious agent, it is useful for respiratory infections, including bronchitis, sinusitis, and sore throats. It can also help to expectorate catarrh in asthma and seems generally helpful in relieving the symptoms of asthma. It is also used in the treatment of urinary infections, including cystitis and urethritis. Its antispasmodic effects can be used for muscular strain and arthritis. As an insecticide it could be used in the treatment of head lice. It can also be used to treat toothache, a single drop applied on a cotton bud. It is a powerful stimulant and therefore should not be used before retiring.

**Cautions:** High concentrations may irritate the skin.

## Cardamom (Elettaria cardamomum)

**Family:** Zingiberaceae

In the same family as Ginger and Galangal, this plant is native to Asia and parts of the Middle East, but is also grows in France and

South America. It has long leaves and yellow flowers with purple tips. The oil is distilled from the pods, which are packed with small black seeds and usually picked before they are ripe (Green Cardamom), although sometimes after they are ripened. The spice is used for cooking in all types of Asian cuisine and now throughout the world. The oil is used in perfumes, and in aromatherapy. It is distilled from the seed to give a beautifully spicy/floral note.

**Constituents:** Monoterpenes (at least 7%); sabinene, myrcene, limonene, and pinene. Monoterpene alcohols (at least 6%); linalol, terpinene-1-ol-4, $\alpha$-terpineol. Sesquiterpenes; zingerberene. Esters (about 40%); linalyl acetate, terpinyl acetate. Oxides; 1,8 cineole (up to 50%).

**Actions:** Tonic, stimulant, stomachic, carminative, antispasmodic, anti-catarrhal, expectorant, anti-infectous, nervine, cephalic, diuretic, sialagogue, and anthelmintic.

**Uses:** Anorexia, weak digestion, dyspepsia, aerophagy, spasmodic colitis, worms, heart problems of nervous origin, bronchitis, cramps, nervous fatigue, and stress.

**Cautions:** Care should be taken for individuals with sensitive skin.

### Carrot Seed (Daucus carota)

**Family:** Apiaceae

Steam distilled from the dried seeds of the Wild Carrot. The oil is yellow to amber in colour and is mainly produced in France. It smells of carrots. An infused oil is also made from the roots and is bright orange in colour. It is traditionally used in skin care. Care should be taken when purchasing the infused oil since it may actually be made from *Tagetes* spp., which have a different therapeutic profile. For more information, see the data on infused oils.

**Constituents:** Monoterpenes; pinene, limonene. Sesquiterpenes; bisabolene, elemene, caryophyllene. Monoterpenols; geraniol. Sesquiterpenols; carotol, daucol. Esters; geranyl acetate.

**Actions:** Anthelmintic, antiseptic, depurative, diuretic, emmenagogue, hepatic, stimulant, tonic, vasodilatory and smooth muscle relaxant.

**Uses:** Gout, ulcers, flatulence, eczema, and psoriasis.

Used for skin conditions, including dermatitis, eczema, psoriasis, and rashes. Also rejuvenating for congested and stressed skin and reputed to help wrinkles. It is also an excellent liver tonic and, therefore, useful for debility and convalescence. Reputed to help anorexia, anaemia, and colic or indigestion related to liver insufficiency. Has been used for absent or painful periods and premenstrual syndrome. It is reputed to aid with the elimination of toxins and therefore can be used for gout, rheumatism, arthritis and water retention or oedema.

Davis (1991) says that it can help strengthen inner vision, particularly at times of doubt or confusion. Carrot Seed oil also clears energy blocks, particularly between the heart and solar plexus chakras.

**Cautions:** None reported.

## Cedarwood, Atlas (Cedrus atlantica)

**Family:** Pinaceae

**Constituents:** Sesquiterpenes (50%); cedrene, himachalane. Sesquiterpenols (30%); atlantol, caryophyllene alcohol, cubenol. Ketones; atlantones.

**Actions:** Antiseptic, astringent, bacteriostatic, cicatrisant, expectorant, fungicide, insect repellent, lipolytic, lymphotonic, mucolytic, phlebotonic, tonic, diuretic, sedative.

**Uses:** Acne, bronchitis, catarrh, cystitis, dysuria, gonorrhoea, pyelitis, respiratory infections, skin diseases, and urinary tract disorders.

Cedar oil is considered by some to be an aphrodisiac—what is certainly true is that it is deeply relaxing. One of the oils which can be used at night-time for respiratory congestion.

It is valuable as a mucolytic oil. Lawless (1992) reports that it is particularly helpful in chronic congestion, such as bronchitis or intractable chest infections. As an antiseptic it can be used for the treatment of urinary tract infections, including cystitis, and for vaginal infections. Cedarwood oil is also used for infections of the skin and scalp, including fungal infections. It can be used for infestations as well (scabies and lice). For treatment of the skin, it has also been used to treat eczema, pruritis, and acne—where it's woody scent may appeal more to men. For the scalp it can help in stress-induced alopecia and in the treatment of dandruff.

Cedarwood has insect-repelling actions and can be used to keep moths at bay. Also, Cedarwood may be used on bed linen to keep away dust mites and bed bugs.

Finally, it is a tonic to the lymphatic and circulatory systems and as such can be used for arteriosclerosis, cellulite, and water retention.

Emotionally, Davis (1991) recommends it for 'emotional catarrh' and states that it is valuable for purification and to strengthen our spirituality and our connections to the spiritual world.

**Cautions:** Avoid in pregnancy and prolonged use—due to ketones. Pigmentation sometimes occurs after using the oil. Occasionally, Cedarwood causes irritation.

## Cedarwood, Himalayan (Cedrus deodora)

Steam distilled from the wood.
**Family:** Pinaceae
  **Constituents:** Sesquiterpenes; $\alpha$ and $\beta$ himachalenes. Sesquiterpenols; himachalol, allo-himachalol. Ketones; $\alpha$ and $\gamma$ atlantones.
  **Actions:** Anti-atherosclerotic, cicatrisant, antiseptic (urinary, pulmonary), antiputrescent, antiseborrheic, aphrodisiac, astringent, diuretic, emollient, expectorant, fungicidal, insecticidal, mucolytic, lipolytic, sedative, lymphatic tonic, nervine, and rejuvenating.
  **Uses:** Boils, wound healing, cellulite, oily skin, acne, fungal infections of the skin, dandruff, alopecia, respiratory infection or congestion, chronic bronchitis and coughs, rheumatism, arthritis, urinary infections, chronic urethritis, vaginitis, cystitis, oedema, sedative to the nervous system, arthritis, headaches, aftershave, antidepressive, and used for meditation and for developing yoga breathing exercises.
  **Cautions:** Avoid for babies and during pregnancy due to ketone content. Probably best avoided for epileptics too. Appears to be non-toxic and well tolerated at normal dilutions, non-irritating, and non-sensitising. *External use only.*

## Chamomile, German (Chamomilla recutita/Matricaria chamomilla/ Matricaria recutita)

Steam distilled from the flowering heads of the annual herb. During the distillation process large quantities of chamazulene are formed, giving the oil its intense navy blue colour and distinctive odour. The blue colour gradually gains a greenish tinge with age. The oil is moderately viscous. An absolute is also produced for the perfumery industry. Also used as a hydrolat.
  **Constituents:** Monoterpenes; limonene, cymene, ocimene. Sesquiterpenes; chamazulene, bisabolene, farnesene, cadinene, copaene,

caryophyllene, muurolene. Sesquiterpenols; bisabolol, spathulenol, farnesol. Oxides; bisabol oxide, bisabolol oxide, epoxy bisabolol, bisabolone oxide, 1,8-cineole. Coumarins: herniarin, ombelliferone (fungicidal). Ethers; dicycloether.

**Actions:** Analgesic, anti-allergic, anti-inflammatory, anti-spasmodic, bactericide, cicatrisant, cholagogue, decongestant, digestive, febrifuge, fungicide, hormonal, immuno-stimulant, sedative, vermifuge, and vulnerary.

**Uses:** The uses of German Chamomile overlap to a large extent with Roman Chamomile. Its anti-inflammatory action makes it valuable for a variety of skin problems, including acne, allergies, eczema, dermatitis, and all skin irritations, including rashes caused by food allergies. I have also found it useful for the treatment of psoriasis. It will reduce all histamine induced responses, including skin responses, hay fever, painful joints, and asthma. Like Roman chamomile, its combination of actions on the CNS and the digestive system make it useful for gastric spasm, ulcers, gastritis, indigestion, and nausea of nervous origin. Price and Price (2007) suggest its use for morning sickness. An excellent remedy for infants (and corresponding ailments in adults)—teething, colic, sleeplessness, rashes, eczema, earache, and nappy rash. Used for all stress-related conditions, including moodiness, headaches, migraine, insomnia, and indigestion. As an anti-inflammatory, Chamomile is invaluable for arthritis, gout, rheumatism, sprains, and muscular pain. Its mild analgesic action will help with many of the above. It has also been suggested for menstrual disturbances and menopausal symptoms, probably because of the support it gives the nervous system, rather than for any hormone-like action. It has been shown to shorten the time it takes for cutaneous burns to heal. Again, increases leucocyte production. Steam inhalations may also be useful for catarrh and asthma. Chamazulene is effective against *Candida albicans* and *Staphylococcus aureus*. It is therefore valuable for the treatment of both thrush and cystitis. Both Roman and German Chamomiles act as vasoconstrictors, helping to reduce thread veins and enlarged capillaries, but this may take several months, and needs to be combined with a reduction in causative factors. On an emotional level very similar to Roman chamomile.

**Cautions:** Occasionally reports of dermatitis in individuals sensitive to Ragweed. Also, some reports of low oral toxicity, when given to various small, furry creatures.

**Note:** *Artemisia arborescens,* or Mugwort is sometimes sold as Blue Chamomile. It contains large amounts of azulene, but also contains large amounts of thujone and borneone. It should definitely be avoided in pregnancy and by individuals with a tendency of epileptic seizures, also with babies and young children. Again, this shows the necessity of knowing that your oils are from the correct botanical species, as if you ask for Blue Chamomile, meaning German, you may end up with this one!

## Chamomile, Maroc/Moroccan (Ormenis mixta/multicaulis, Anthemis mixta)

Distilled from the flowering herb, this essential oil is mobile and a yellow or brown colour, *definitely not blue!* Morocco is the main area of distillation.

**Constituents:** Monoterpenes:; $\alpha$-pinene, camphene, limonene, terpinene, terpinolene. Sesquiterpenes; germacrene, $\beta$-caryophyllene, bisabolene, $\alpha$-elemene. Monoterpenols; terpineol, linalol, borneol, ormenol, trans-pinocarveol, santolina, yomogi, and artemisia alcohols. Ketones; borneone and pinocamphone. Oxides; 1,8-cineole. Esters; bornyl acetate and bornyl butanoate.

**Actions:** Anti-infectious, bactericide, hepatic, parasiticide, neurotonic, tonic, and tonic to the reproductive system (both male and female).

This oil is primarily an anti-infectious oil, being particularly effective against *E. coli.* This makes it useful for cystitis and other problems caused by this bacterium. It is also effective against intestinal parasites, including round worms and amoebae. It is a tonic to the liver and digestive system, also the pancreas. It is also used for dry and itchy skin conditions, including eczema of that description. Other applications include nervous depression, atherosclerosis, and prostatitis. As an anti-infectious oil, it can also be used for acne, abscesses, and cysts.

**Cautions:** The main constituents are a terpene and an alcohol, thus there is little need for caution at normal doses. However, the presence of ketones mean that it is probably best to avoid this during pregnancy and that it should not be used for long periods of time without a break.

## Chamomile, Roman (Chamemelum nobile/Anthemis nobilis)

**Family:** Asteraceae

The oil is distilled from the flowering tops of the plant. The fresh oil is almost imperceptibly yellow/blue and the colour deepens with age to a darker blue green. The colour is very faint, unlike German chamomile. The oil has an apple/banana aroma due to the high content of esters. The main areas of production are England, Belgium, Hungary, USA, Italy, and France. A hydrolat is also produced and has wide therapeutic applications.

**Constituents:** Monoterpenes; α-terpene, α-pinene, β-pinene, sabinene, camphene, myrcene, terpinene, cymene. Sesquiterpenes; sabinene, caryophyllene, chamazulene, copaene, cadinene. Monoterpenols; pino carveol. Sesquiterpenols; farnesol and nerolidol. Aldehydes; myrtenal. Ketones; pinocarvone. Esters (75–80%); angelic and tiglic acids. Oxides; 1,8-cineole. Coumarins; trace.

**Actions:** Analgesic, anti-anaemic, anti-inflammatory, anti-parasitic, antiseptic, antispasmodic, bactericidal, calming, carminative, cholagogue, cicatrisant, digestive, emmenagogue, febrifuge, hepatic, hypnotic, immuno-stimulant, nerve sedative, ophthalmic, stomachic, sudorific, tonic, vermifuge, and vulnerary.

**Uses:** The high levels of esters in this oil make it an excellent antispasmodic and nerve tonic. Thus, it is applied for migraine, headaches, and diarrhoea (especially of nervous origin), and its hepatic action helps in all these areas. Its digestive and hepatic actions make it useful for flatulence, colic in adults and children, indigestion, and loss of appetite. Irritable bowel and colitis also seem to respond well to this oil (my personal observation). Its calming action also make it valuable for the treatment of insomnia, depression, and stress-induced moodiness and irritability. It is also indicated for shock in some texts. Whilst it can be valuable for post shock recovery, true shock is potentially life threatening and should probably be attended to by a doctor. Actions as a CNS regulator and on the female reproductive system make it a valuable oil for menstrual and menopausal mood disturbances and it would appear to help amenorrhoea and dysmenorrhoea also. Chamomile tea has been traditionally used for cystitis and urinary problems. As an anti-inflammatory, the oil can be used for a wide range of conditions; eczema, dermatitis, urticaria and other skin irritations, cracked nipples, teething and inflamed gums in infants and adults, irritation or conjunctivitis of the eye, rheumatism, and gout. The oil may also be used for sensitive skin and the treatment of boils, burns and cuts or grazes. Lastly, Chamomile oil appears to promote the production of both healthy white and red blood cells, this means that it can help in the treatment of anaemia and of lowered immunity. It has this in common with Lemon (*Citrus limomum*).

On an emotional level, Chamomile is said to induce a more positive frame of mind, and is definitely an excellent sedative and calmer of the nerves.

According to Patricia Davis (1991) this oil has an affinity to the throat chakra, and should be used when there are problems with communication. It responds to the higher vibrations of this centre and allows communication of spiritual truths. She also recommends it for overactivity of any centre, anger, redness, and heat.

**Cautions:** Although widely used for allergic conditions in sensitised individuals, it may cause allergic responses; therefore, it is wise to use patch testing before using any oil on a hypersensitive individual. Particularly reported to cause sensitisation in individuals allergic to Ragweed (*Senecio jacobea*).

## Cinnamon Leaf (Cinnamomum zeylanicum)

**Family:** Lauraceae

Oil is steam distilled from the leaves. An oil is also distilled from the bark to use in perfumery and is not suitable for use in practice as it is a powerful skin irritant due to content of cinnamaldehyde. The leaf oil smells more like cloves.

**Constituents:** Phenols (80–96%); eugenol. Aldehydes; cinnamaldehyde (3%). Esters; eugenol acetate and bensyl benzoate. Alcohols; linalool. Phenyl ethers; safrol.

**Actions:** Antiseptic, antiputrescent, antispasmodic, cardiac stimulant, emmenagogue, haemostatic, and parasiticide.

**Uses:** Bruises, colds, colitis, contusions, convalescence, debility, diarrhoea, fainting, flatulence, flu, frigidity, gastric infections, gastric pain and spasm, haemoptysis, impotence, intestinal parasites, leucorrhoea, menstrual problems, putrefactive fermentations, scanty menstrual periods, sluggish digestion, toothache, uterine haemorrhage, wasp stings. Cinnamon tea for elderly people and to protect against flus and infections, lice, scabies, warts, poor circulation, debility, and nervous exhaustion. Cinnamon leaf oil masks the smell of cigarette smoke.

**Cautions:** Prolonged use as hepatotoxic, skin irritant. Do not use in pregnancy.

## Cistus, Labdanum (Cistus ladanifer)

**Family:** Cistaceae

A bush or shrub native to the dry, rocky regions of the Mediterranean, especially Crete and Cyprus, but also grown in Spain. It has beautiful white flowers and can be grown as an ornamental in these regions. The branches are now used to steam distil a viscous dark brown oil. Cistus has beautiful white flowers and the leaves exude a resin, known as labdanum. The oil is now distilled from the branches, to give a viscous resinous, dark brown oil. The oil was formerly prepared from resin gathered from the wool of sheep and goats grazing on the hillsides.

**Constituents:** Monoterpenes; $\alpha$-pinene, camphene. Alcohols; borneol (2%). Diterpene; labdane-8-$\alpha$-15-diol, acetoxy-15-labdanol-8. Esters; linalyl acetate, bornyl acetate, methyl benzoates, benzyl benzoates, phenyl methyl phenylippropanaote, ethyl pinoate, ethyl gamma campholenates. Phenols; eugenol (1%), thymol. Ketones; 2,2,6 trimethylcyclohexanone (2%), fenchone (1%). Acetophenones (1.5%). Acids (1.8%). Lactones; bicyclobutyrolactone, tuberolactone, and 12-nor-ambreinolide.

**Actions:** Anti-infectious, antiviral, antibacterial, antihaemorrhagic, cicatrisant, anti-arthritis, neurotonic, and nervine.

**Uses:** Childhood illnesses—chickenpox, scarlet fever etc., viral infections and autoimmune disease, haemorrhages of the rectum and colon, polyarthritis and rheumatism, insomnia, and nervousness. It also has a reputation for helping to heal past life traumas and for working with rituals.

## Clary Sage (Salvia sclarea)

**Family:** Labiatae/Lamiaceae

There are over 250 constituents in Clary Sage oil, which is why it is often cited as containing top, middle, and base notes. It is cultivated in France, Russia, USA, Morocco, and central Europe, and the flowering tops are the part used for oil. Extracted by steam distillation, pale yellow with a green tinge or sometimes colourless. The smell is musky and nutty. Generally appreciated by men.

**Constituents:** Monoterpenes; α-pinene, β-pinene, sabinene, camphene, myrcene, terpinolene, para-cymene, terpinene, limonene. Sesquiterpenes; β-caryophyllene, germacrene, curcumene, trans-calamene, trans-ocimene, terpinolene, cubene, α-copaene, β-bourbonene. Monoterpenols (15%); linalol, ∂-terpineol, citronellol, nerol, geraniol, borneol, thujol, terpineol-4. Sesquiterpenols; bisabol, junerol. Diterpenols; sclareol (1–7%). Aldehydes; hexanal, caryophenal. Esters; linalyl acetate (49–75%), citronellyl acetate, geranyl acetate, neryl acetate, butryates, valerates, bornyl acetate, terpinyl acetate. Oxides; 1,8-cineole, linalol oxide, caryophyllene oxide, sclareol oxide. Ketones; trace of thujone. Coumarin.

**Actions:** Anti-infectious, anti-convulsive, antidepressant, antifungal, antispasmodic, astringent, anti-sudorific, bactericidal, carminative, digestive, decongestant, detoxicant, emmenagogue, euphoric, hypotensor, oestrogen-like, nervine, phlebotonic, regenerative, sedative, tonic.

**Uses:** One of the oils with an action on the female reproductive system. Clary sage is particularly useful for spasms in this system, including painful periods and to ease delivery by encouraging smooth contractions. It can also be used to encourage the onset of menstruation. However, overuse can make menstruation excessively heavy. If being used for regulation restrict its use to the first two weeks of the cycle. It can also be used to treat vaginal infections because of hormonal imbalance. Indicated for the symptoms of menopause, particularly hot flushes and night sweats. As an antispasmodic it also has an affinity to the digestive system, and can be used for colic, stomach cramps, dyspepsia, and flatulence. For the respiratory system it is indicated for asthma where both its antispasmodic and nervine actions come into play. Also used for throat infections and laryngitis. As a circulatory tonic, it can be used to treat varicose veins, haemorrhoids, and may be useful for aneurysms. It also lowers blood pressure and cholesterol. In skin care it is indicated for acne and boils, especially where there is hormonal imbalance, and is used for both oily and aging skin. Reputed to arrest hair loss and banish dandruff. Also used to treat fungal skin infections. For the nervous system it can help alleviate depression, tension, and stress-related problems and is particularly useful for debility in convalescence. Clary Sage is indicated for migraine and sexual difficulties including frigidity and impotence. Other uses include epilepsy and muscular spasm. It has also been used with success in the treatment of arthritic pain. Davis (1991) says that this oil brings us in touch with the dream world and helps us to see more clearly with our inner eye.

**Cautions:** Probably best avoided in pregnancy. Those with low blood pressure should use it with caution. Do not use if operating heavy machinery or driving, due to it's euphoric and hypnotic actions. Does not mix well with alcohol—the two combined can cause lurid dreams.

## Clove Bud (Eugenia caryophyllus/Syzgium aromaticum)

**Family:** Myrtaceae

The oil is steam distilled from the buds. It is a pale-yellow colour. Mainly produced in Madagascar and Indonesia. It is interesting to note that the original wild trees found in the Molucca Islands do not yield any eugenol.

**Constituents:** Monoterpenes; pinenes. Sesquiterpenes; caryophyllenes, humulene cubebene, copaene. Phenols (60–90%); eugenol. Esters (20–25%); linalyl acetate, nonanal acetate, terpinyl acetate, benzyl acetate, methyl benzoate. Oxides; mululene epoxide caryophyllene oxide.

**Actions:** Analgesic due to eugenol, anti-infectious, antifungal, antiviral, antiseptic, antispasmodic, calming, carminative, cicatrisant, hypertensor, immuno-stimulant, insect repellent, mental stimulant, nervine, stimulant, parasiticide, uterine tonic. Possibly anti-cancer.

**Uses:** An oil that is best treated with caution due to its dermal toxicity and cumulative effects. However, invaluable as a fumigant to keep respiratory infections at bay. It has a strong analgesic action, which can benefit conditions including toothache, rheumatoid arthritis, and neuralgia. It is used for gastrointestinal infections and wind or spasm in the intestines, also diarrhoea. Also used for gum infections and abscesses, but dilute well before use to prevent local haemorrhage. Its antiseptic action can also be used for salpingitis, pulmonary infections, and infected skin conditions, such as acne, infected wounds, and ulcers. Clove bud oil also boosts the immune system and can be used for influenza, herpes, hepatitis, and tuberculosis. An excellent oil for getting rid of creeping creatures, including flies, moths, and scabies mites. It can be used in labour for its analgesic effects and to facilitate delivery. A stimulating oil which can benefit fatigue, general debility, and memory loss. Clove bud oil also promotes the secretion of saliva and can balance the thyroid gland.

**Cautions:** Clove bud oil is a skin irritant and prolonged use can cause liver damage. High concentrations may cause local haemorrhage. Avoid in pregnancy but can be used in labour. Oils distilled from the stem or leaf should not be used since they can cause severe skin irritation and can be sensitisers.

## Cypress (Cupressus sempervirens)

**Family:** Cupressaceae

Steam distilled from the twigs and branchlets. Mainly produced in France, Spain, and Morocco. The oil is yellow to olive green. A concrete and absolute are also produced in small amounts.

**Constituents:** Monoterpenes (80%); pinenes, camphene, carene, limonene, terpinolene, cymene, sabinene, terpinene. Sesquiterpenes; cedrene, cadinene, ocimenes. Monoterpenols; terpineol-4, $\alpha$-terpineol, borneol, linalol, sabinol. Sesquiterpenols; cedrol. Diterpenols; manool, abienol, pimarinol, toarol. Oxides; 1,8-cineole, manoyl oxide. Esters; terpenyl acetate, terpinenyl-4 acetate.

**Actions:** Anti-infectious, antispasmodic, anti-sudorific, astringent, antitussive, astringent, antibacterial, calming, circulatory tonic, deodorant, diuretic, neurotonic, sedative, phlebotonic, hormonal action, vasoconstrictor.

**Uses:** This oil is a very valuable astringent and many of its uses are due, in part, to this property. As a pectoral (lung tonic) it is used to treat bronchitis, flu, whooping cough, spasmodic coughs, and emphysema. It can also be helpful in the treatment of asthma.

For the circulatory system it is a vasoconstrictor, which means it can be used to relieve varicose veins, haemorrhoids and thread veins or broken capillaries. In fact, any condition where the blood is breaking through the vessels since it is a tonic to the venous and capillary circulation. It can also help where there is excess fluid or oedema. It can also be used where there is see page through the skin from severe oedema. However, caution should be exercised if there is hypertension due to its constrictive action on the blood vessels.

Due to the terpene content, Cypress is generally good for drying excess fluid and therefore can be used for excessive perspiration, including sweaty feet and night sweats experienced in menopause or various fevers. During menopause it has a hormonal action that will also help relieve other symptoms. This also helps with dysmenorrhoea and with excessively heavy periods. Other damp conditions it can help with are rheumatic inflammation and diarrhoea, also incontinence and enuresis. It is a nervine and therefore can relieve exhaustion, nervous tension, and irritability. Here its anti-infectious action helps to support a stressed immune system and its action on the liver helps to reduce physiological stress and various liver problems. It is also valuable for pet care and skin care. Emotionally, Cypress has a long association with death and the afterlife. It is therefore considered to be strengthening at the time of death and to help with major transitions in life.

### Elemi/Manila Elemi/Java Almond (Canarium luzonicum)

**Family:** Burseraceae

From the gum-resin exudate of a tree native to the Philippines and South America, Elemi has been used in Europe for 500 years in salves and liniments.

**Constituents:** Sesquiterpenes; elemens. Monoterpenes; $\alpha$ and $\beta$ phellandrenes (15 and 7%) limonene, terpiolene, pinene, dipentene. Sesquiterpenols; elemol, terpineol, carvone.

**Actions:** Astringent, anti-inflammatory, analgesic, possibly antiviral, antiseptic, anti-amoebic, balsamic, cicatrisant, expectorant, fungicidal, stimulant, vulnerary.

**Uses:** Inflammation, respiratory conditions, nerves, muscles, lymph, joints, wounds, congestion, bleeding in skin, aged skin, rejuvenation, wrinkles, chronic conditions of the skin, fungal infections, varicose ulcers, gangrene, strengthens the immune system, diarrhoea, dyspepsia, may stimulate the thymus, nervous exhaustion, stress-related conditions. Supposedly grounding, instils joy and peace, centring, and is balancing of the upper and lower chakras.

**Cautions:** May cause skin irritation, so use at low concentrations.

### Eucalyptus (Eucalyptus spp.)

**Family:** Myrtaceae

### Eucalyptus globulus

The oil is obtained from the leaves of the tree by steam distillation, the oil from mature and immature leaves differing in composition. The tree is native to Australia but is also cultivated in China, Spain, and Portugal. The oil is virtually colourless and very fluid. The main route of elimination is via the lungs, making it valuable in treating respiratory conditions. The majority of eucalyptus oil is rectified, even that supplied to the aromatherapy trade. It is, therefore, desirable to use an organically produced oil and one that is unrectified. You should check this with your supplier. Unrectified eucalyptus oil has a far softer and more rounded aroma, with fruity and almost floral undertones.

**Constituents:** Monoterpenes; pinene, cymene limonene, camphene. Sesquiterpenes; aromadendrene, phellandrene. Monoterpenols; fenchyl alcohol, terpineol, myrtenol. Sesquiterpenols; globulol, ledol, trans-pinocarveol, viridiflorol. Ketones; pinocarvone, carvone, fenchone, Oxides; 1,8-cineole, pinene epoxide. Aldehydes; myrtenal, geranial, valeric aldehyde, butyric aldehyde, caproic aldehyde. Esters; terpenyl acetate.

**Actions:** Analgesic, antifungal, anti-infectious, anti-inflammatory, antiseptic, anti-viral, antibacterial, balsamic, decongestant, deodorant, depurative, diuretic, expectorant, insect repellent, mucolytic, rubefacient, stimulant, vulnerary.

**Uses:** Respiratory infections, including acute bronchitis, flu, pneumonia, pleurisy, sinusitis, laryngitis, colds where it's balsamic property also acts to reduce fever. Also coughs and asthma. As an anti-infectious oil, it is also used for cystitis and other urinary tract infections, and the treatment of candida. Its decongesting actions are used in the treatment of migraine and headaches. As a rubefacient and anti-inflammatory it is used in the relief of arthritis and rheumatism and may also be used for muscular aches and pains. Eucalyptus' healing actions are used in the treatment of burns. As an anti-viral, it is effective against herpes, shingles, cold sores, measles, and scarlet fever. As a bactericide it is effective against staphylococcal infections and can be used as a fumigant to prevent infection spreading. Being strongly stimulant, it is not recommended for evening use unless blended with a relaxing oil at higher concentration.

Another use for Eucalyptus is as a grease dissolving agent, excellent for removing tar and oil stains.

**Cautions:** Contraindicated for small babies and children, due to ketone content; therefore, best to avoid in pregnancy also. Several cases of intestinal irritation, leading to fatality reported, therefore best avoided orally. Prolonged use should be avoided. Large doses will also irritate the kidneys.

## Eucalyptus citriodora

**Constituents:** Monoterpenes; pinene. Monoterpenols; citronellol, geraniol. Aldehydes; citronellal. Esters: citronyl acetate.

**Actions:** Analgesic, anti-inflammatory, antiseptic, antispasmodic, anti-viral, bactericidal, circulatory tonic, deodorant, expectorant, fungicidal, insecticide, sedative.

**Uses:** Its strong anti-inflammatory action makes it particularly valuable for all forms of arthritis and rheumatism. It is also useful for treating other inflammations of the soft connective tissues, including tendinitis and bursitis conditions (e.g. tennis elbow, golfer's elbow, housemaid's knee etc.). It is also used for hypertension. As an antiseptic it is used for vaginal infections and cystitis. It can also be used for shingles. The aldehyde content makes *Eucalyptus citriodora* a valuable antifungal to treat athlete's foot and other fungal infections. It is particularly effective against infections of *Staphylococcus aureus*, due to synergy between the citronellol and citronellal. It may also be used as an insect repellent and in the treatment of dandruff.

**Cautions:** The high level of aldehydes mean that there is the potential for dermal irritation and sensitisation. Therefore, use at low concentrations and only for three weeks before alternating with another oil.

## Eucalyptus dives

**Constituents:** Monoterpenes; $\alpha$-phellandrene (30%). Sesquiterpenes; $\alpha$-cubebene, $\beta$-caryophyllene, longifolene, elemene, cadinene. Monoterpenols; linalol, terpineol-4, $\alpha$-terpineol, piperitol. Ketones; piperitone (40–50%).

**Actions:** Anti-infectious, antibacterial, diuretic, renal regenerant, mucolytic.

**Uses:** Used for upper respiratory infections, including sinusitis, otitis, and bronchitis. Also used for catarrhal congestion. It's affinity for the urinary system makes it useful for nephritis, and urinary infections. It is also useful for leucorrhoea, arthritis, rheumatism, aches, pains, and sports injuries. Also indicated for headaches, neuralgia, and sciatica.

**Cautions:** High in ketones, therefore do not used in pregnancy or on infants under six years old.

## Eucalyptus polybractea

**Constituents:** Monoterpenes; paracymene (30%). Monterpenols; linalol, terpineol-4, α-terpineol. Sesquiterpenols; eudesmol. Aldehydes; myrtenal, geranial, cuminal, phellandral. Ketones: cryptone (40%), piperitone. Oxides; 1,8-cineole.

**Actions:** Anticatarrhal, anti-infectious, antibacterial, antiviral, anti-inflammatory, expectorant, healing, lipolytic, mucolytic.

**Uses:** Prostatitis. It is also used for respiratory infections, especially pharyngitis, bronchitis, and for asthma. It is a useful anti-inflammatory for arthritis.

**Cautions:** Its high ketone levels mean that it should not be used in pregnancy, babies, or small infants.

## Eucalyptus radiata

*Eucalyptus radiata* contains practically no components that could be regarded as ketones and, therefore, can be liberally applied as an expectorant. However, *Eucalyptus globulus* contains pinocarvone and is therefore appropriately used in lower concentrations as a mucolytic.

**Constituents:** Monoterpenes; pinenes, myrcene. Monoterpenols (20%); linalol, borneol, terpineol-4, geraniol. Aldehydes; myrtenal, citronellal, geranial, neral. Oxides; 1,8-cineole (62–72%).

**Actions:** Anti-infectious, antibacterial, antiviral, anti-inflammatory, expectorant.

**Uses:** Flu, sinusitis, bronchitis, otitis, coughs, acne This oil is particularly quick at penetrating.

**Cautions:** A safe form of Eucalyptus, with no contraindications, if used at normal doses.

## Eucalyptus smithii

**Constituents:** Monoterpenes; limonene, pinene, paracymene. Monoterpenols; terpineol, terpineol-4, geraniol, linalool. Sesquiterpenols; eudesmol. Oxides; 1,8-cineole. Esters; small quantities. Aldehyde; isovaleraldehyde.

**Actions:** Analgesic, anti-infectious, anticatarrhal, antiviral, balancing, decongestant, digestif, expectorant, immunostimulant.

**Uses:** Again, used for the respiratory tract, particularly as an expectorant. Its mucolytic actions are negligible since it contains no ketones. It is therefore more like the E. *radiata* type. A blend of this with E. *radiata* is particularly useful for fluidifying mucus and expectorating. If a terpene rich oil, such as one of the pines, is added, the effect is even better.

**Cautions:** No specific known. Makes a useful active excipient in frictions, especially for respiratory problems.

## Sweet Fennel (Foeniculum vulgare var. dulce)

**Family:** Apiaceae

Steam distilled from the crushed seeds of sweet fennel. Bitter fennel oil is not appropriate for use.

**Constituents:** Monoterpenes; pinene, limonene, phellandrene, thujene, camphene, sabinene, myrcene, terpinene, ocimene. Monoterpenols; fenchol (3–4%). Ketones; d-fenchone (0–22%). Phenyl ethers; methyl chavicol (2–12%), cis-anethole (0–1.7%), trans-anethole (50–90%). Aldehydes; anisaldehyde (0–0.5%). Oxides; 1,8-cineole (1–6%). Coumarins; bergaptene, umbelliferone.

**Actions:** Analgesic, anti-inflammatory, antiseptic, antispasmodic, antitoxic, aperitif, carminative, cardiotonic, cholagogue, choleretic, circulatory stimulant, digestive, diuretic, emmenagogue, expectorant, galactogogue, laxative, litholytic, oestrogen-like, respiratory tonic, splenetic, stomachic, tonic, urinary tract antiseptic.

**Uses:** An oil that people love or hate due to the 'aniseed' aroma, which also makes it difficult to blend aesthetically. However, small amounts can be gorgeous (try fennel and cinnamon). Fennel's main therapeutic indications are for it's oestrogen-like, digestive, and diuretic effects.

Fennel oil is traditionally thought of as detoxifying. It has been traditionally used against snake bites, but you are unlikely to come across such casualties here. However, the detoxifying effect can be of benefit for recovering alcoholics, where it's action on the liver also plays a part. These effects are also useful after slight overindulgences. Also indicated for arthritis, cellulite, oedema, gout, and probably helpful for rheumatoid arthritis due to its hormonal action.

The hormonal action also means that it can help regularise the female cycle. Along with Clary Sage it should be used up to ovulation to help bring this into line. Fennel also relieves the symptoms of menopause and premenstrual syndrome. Should be avoided in pregnancy but can be used after to encourage the flow of milk. In this instance, it is probably best to use in the form of a tea made from the whole herb. This will also help any colic in the infant. Also indicated for constipation, flatulence, nausea, and indigestion, especially where liver hypofunction seems to be the cause. It appears to normalise the appetite and therefore can help with certain types of obesity.

As a diuretic it can relieve cellulite, kidney problems, and urinary stones. It is also a mild analgesic so can be used for backache, painful periods, bruises, gum infections, and painful menstruation.

Also indicated for palpitations and over rapid breathing, partly due to its effect on the nervous system. Davis (1991) says that it is traditionally used to protect from evil or witches and, therefore, may be useful when feeling under psychic attack.

**Cautions:** Do not use in pregnancy. Avoid in epilepsy and for children under six years of age. Also avoid prolonged use.

## Frankincense (Boswellia carterii/thurifera)

**Family:** Burseraceae

Frankincense is widely used in religious ceremonies. Take care to get the distilled oil, rather than a solvent extracted resinoid. The gum is often mixed with those from other trees called Frankincense e.g. *B. bhau-dajana, B. papyifera, B. sacra, B. serrata*. Since the Frankincense forests are under threat, only buy from sustainable sources. *Boswellia serrata* is native to India; *B. papyrifera* is native to Ethiopia and *B. carterii* is from Puntland or north eastern Somalia. The resins are harvested from wild forests in these regions, normally by local villagers.

**Constituents:** Monoterpenes (40%); $\alpha$-pinene, camphene, limonene, dipentene, myrcene, terpinene, thujene, para-cymene, sabinene, phellandrene, terpinolene. Sesquiterpenes; caryophyllene, gurjunene, guaiene, copaene. Alcohols; borneol, terpineol-4, pinocarveol, farnesone. Ketones; verbenone. Esters; octyl acetate. Ketone alcohol; olibanol. Alcohol oxide; incenseoloxide.

**Actions:** Analgesic, anti-inflammatory, antidepressant, antioxidant, antiseptic, astringent, cicatrisant, cytophylactic, digestive, diuretic, emmenagogue, expectorant, immunomodulant, sedative, tonic, uterine tonic, vulnerary.

**Uses:** Anxiety, breast inflammations, catarrh, colds, coughs, cystitis, depression, dysmenorrhoea, flus, laryngitis, lethargy, meditation, metrorrhagia, nephritis, rheumatism, skin care, ulcers, varicose veins, varicose ulcers, wounds.

Used for skincare, particularly dry, mature, and ageing skin and also for pimples, scars, ulcers, wounds, reputed to smooth oil wrinkles, antiseptic tonic to all skin, and balances oily skin.

Soothing for bronchitis, asthmatic and catarrhal pleurisy, laryngitis, excess mucus, eases shortness of breath, slows and deepens breathing.

Anxiety, nervous tension, depression, stress, post-traumatic shock, nightmares, fear of future, indecision. It produces calm, soothed, elevated mental states, used for obsessional states and ties with past blocking growth, brings peace, strengthens beliefs, eternal divine connection, cleans aura and psychic planes. Seems to soothe the mind, but also stimulate clear thought. Reputed to be helpful to people who tend to live in the past or who are trying to overcome old traumas.

**Cautions:** None reported in regards to toxicity or side effects, though some recommend it is avoided in pregnancy due to unknown constituents. However, due to the overuse, harvesting, and various other factors, we really need to question whether we need to use this oil or whether we can use something else instead. I find Elemi a good alternative for many of its actions.

## Geranium (Pelargonium graveolens/Pelargonium x asperum)

**Family:** Geraniaceae

Obtained by steam distillation from the leaves. The oil is produced in Reunion/Bourbon, Egypt, Russia, and China. The colour of the oil and its chemical constitution will vary with the region of cultivation. The Bourbon type is the most expensive and is a deep olive green clear liquid. The Egyptian and Chinese are pale yellowish green. The chemical composition varies according to the country of origin. An absolute and concrete are produced in Morocco. A floral water is also available.

**Constituents:** Aldehydes (Bourbon) (<10%); neral, geranial combined (<9%), citronellal. Esters (15%); citronellyl formates, geranyl formates, citronellyl proprionates, geranyl proprionates, geranyl tiglates, geranyl acetates, citronellyl butryrate, geranyl acetate, citronellyl butryrate, geranyl butryrate, phenyl ethyl butryrate, phenyl ethyl tiglate. Ketones (1–8%); menthone, iso-menthone, piperitone, methyl heptanone, furopelargone. Oxides; cis-rose oxide, trans-rose oxide, cis-linalol oxide, trans linalol oxide. Alcohols (55–65%); citronellol, geraniol, linalol, nerol, $\alpha$-terpineol, 10-epi-g-eudesmol phenyl ethyl alcohol. Monoterpenes; $\alpha$-phellandrene, $\beta$-phellandrene, $\alpha$-pinene, $\beta$-pinene, myrcene, limonene, cis-ocimene. Sesquiterpenes; guaia-6,9-diene, guaiazulene, $\alpha$-copaene, d-cadinene, t-cadinene, $\alpha$-bourbonene, $\beta$-borbonene.

**Actions:** Analgesic, antidiabetic, anti-infectious, anti-inflammatory, antifungal, antiseptic, antispasmodic, astringent, antibacterial, cicatrisant, deodorant, decongestant, digestive stimulant, fungicidal, haemostatic, insect repellent, relaxant, phlebotonic, styptic, vermifuge, vulnerary.

**Uses:** Traditionally Geranium is used in skin care and balancing both the moods and the hormones. Geranium is applied in skin care for acne, burns, cuts, ulcers (mouth and varicose), and stretch marks. It may also be helpful for dermatitis and dry eczema, although used cautiously in these conditions as some individuals may display sensitivity. I have also used it in the treatment of psoriasis. Its antifungal actions can be useful in the treatment of athlete's foot, nail fungus, and other fungal skin disorders, as well as candida. It may also be indicated in the treatment of impetigo. As an insect repellent, it has been cited as repelling gnats and mosquitoes and getting rid of lice. It seems to balance fluid levels in the body and may help in the treatment of kidney stones. It's action on the circulation and lymphatic system include the treatment of varicose veins, haemorrhoids, water retention, cellulite, and breast and lymphatic congestion. It may also be used in the treatment of uterine haemorrhage and excessively heavy periods. As a balancer of the hormonal system, Geranium oil has been cited for it's action on the pancreas, possibly regulating insulin production. It also may regulate the adrenal cortex and the liver. It also seems to regulate the mood swings associated with PMS and menopause and may help with painful periods. Other indications include rheumatism, osteo-arthritis, pruritis, tonsillitis, and colitis. On an emotional level, geranium is above all relaxing and balancing. Its effect by vaporisation in a fraught atmosphere can be quite remarkable and in states of agitation and anxiety it is excellent. Due to its action on the adrenal cortex, it is also useful for debility, stress, and nervous exhaustion. On the psyche it is claimed to dispel anger and its green colour and pink flowers would indicate a special affinity to the heart chakra. It's distribution of constituents suggest it to be especially indicative for linking the higher and lower chakras and clearing blocks around the solar plexus area.

**Cautions:** Some hypersensitive individuals have experienced dermatitis when used on the skin. Due to its hormone balancing actions, it may be better to avoid in early pregnancy. It contains in excess of 350 constituents and, therefore, has a complex aroma that some find unpleasant when first introduced to the oils.

### Ginger (Zingiber officinalis)

**Family:** Zingiberaceae

Steam distilled from the unpeeled dried root. Heating causes the production of a component particularly useful for the treatment of nausea. The oil smells similar to fresh ginger and is a green-yellow colour.

**Constituents:** Monoterpenes (20%); pinene, camphene, myrcene, limonene, phellandrene. Sesquiterpenes (55%); zingiberene, $\beta$-sesquiphellandrene, curcumene, bisabolene, copaene, sesquithujene, $\beta$-ylangene, $\beta$-elemene, $\beta$-farnesene, $\beta$-caryophyllene, calamenene, $\beta$-bisabolene, selinene. Alcohols; citronellol, linalol, butanol, nonanol, heptanol, nerolidol, elemol, bisabol, zingiberol, trans-$\beta$-sesquiphellandrol, gingerol, borneol. Aldehydes; citronellal, myrtenal, phellandral, neral, geranial. Oxides; 1,8-cineole.

**Actions:** Analgesic, antiseptic, carminative, decongestant, expectorant, febrifuge, laxative, rubefacient, stimulant, stomachic, tonic.

**Uses:** To my mind, an underused oil with many applications. It is a warming stimulant used in Chinese medicine for cold, damp conditions, which makes ideal for use in the Irish climate. As a fumigant it keeps germs at bay. It can be used to treat chills, colds, fevers, and flus. Also, for catarrh and chronic bronchitis. This may be in the form of the oil or as a tea made from the dried Ginger with lemon and/or honey. Also, for sore throats and tonsillitis. The tea may also be drunk to help improve circulation.

**Cautions:** Skin irritation—use at low concentrations.

### Immortelle, Everlasting (Helichrysum italicum/angustifolium)

**Family:** Asteraceae

Steam distilled from the fresh flowers and flowering tops of the plant, which is related to the species widely grown in horticulture. An absolute is also produced by solvent extraction. The oil is yellow to red, with a fresh green odour. Lawless (1992) describes it as honey-like with a tea-like undertone. Mainly cultivated in Spain, Italy, France, and Yugoslavia.

**Constituents:** Sesquiterpenes; $\beta$-caryophyllene. Monoterpenols; nerol. Esters; neryl acetate (75%), neryl butyrate. Ketones; $\beta$-diones, italidones (15–20%).

**Actions:** Anticoagulant, antiphlebitis, antihaematoma, hypocholesterolemic, liver regenerating, anticatarrhal, mucolytic, expectorant, antispasmodic, cicatrisant.

**Uses:** Another under-rated oil. The true oil is expensive, but dramatic in action. It is excellent for the treatment of bruising and haematomas. I have seen it used on severe bruising with rapid results. Also, on older haematomas with good results. Immortelle may also be used on old scars, wounds, couperose, and thread veins. It is reported to be helpful for phlebitis and has been used for the treatment of thromboses. The respiratory actions combine with these healing actions in the treatment of haemoptysis, where I have also seen good results. Immortelle is indicative for rhinitis, bronchitis, spasmodic coughing, and whooping cough. It's action on the liver makes it helpful for any hepatic insufficiency, particularly under stress and in convalescence. It can be helpful for headaches of hepatic origin and viral colitis. Indicated for arthritis. I have used it in the treatment of eczema, psoriasis and dermatitis with good results. It is also helpful for depression and nervous exhaustion.

On an energetic level, Davis (1991) uses the oil for stimulating the right hemisphere of the brain. This allows us to use the creative and intuitive part of ourselves. It is also said to encourage compassion. I have used it to heal old wounds in the psyche.

**Cautions:** Some controversy, since some authorities say that italidiones are *non-toxic* ketones, whilst others say that the same cautions apply.

## Juniper Berries Juniperus communis

**Family:** Cupressaceae

Steam distilled from the berries which take two years to ripen. The oil is colourless or pale yellow and is said to give the urine a scent of violets. The berries are traditionally used to spring clean the system. Savin oil comes from a related species and is highly toxic, make sure you are getting the correct oil. Principle area of production Croatia.

An oil is distilled from the leaves and branchlets with antiseptic, diuretic and anti-rheumatic Actions and is used for bronchitis, anti-catarrh, expectorant. It also facilitates acid excretion via the kidneys.

**Constituents:** Monoterpenes (60–80%); pinenes, limonene, camphene, thujene, sabinene, myrcene, terpinene, cymene, carene, terpinolene, phellandrenes, tolylpropene, cubebene, dimethylstyrene. Sesquiterpenes; $\beta$-caryophyllene, copaene, cadinene, humulene, germacrene. Monoterpenols; terpineol-4 (2–10%), borneol, geraniol. Sesquiterpenols; elemol, eudesmol, cadinol. Oxides; caryophyllene oxide. Esters; bornyl acetate, terpinyl acetate. Coumarins; umbelliferone.

**Actions:** Analgesic, antiseptic, antispasmodic, antitoxic, astringent, carminative, depurative, digestive tonic, diuretic, emmenagogue, hepatic tonic, nervine, pancreatic tonic, parasiticide, rubefacient, sedative, tonic, vulnerary,

**Uses:** Juniper oil is noted for its cleansing actions, particularly eliminating via the kidneys. This makes it a valuable oil in the treatment of cystitis, but caution should be taken where the kidneys are inflamed, since is diuretic action appears to be due to irritating the kidneys. It may also be used in the treatment of kidney stones. As Juniper encourages water to be passed, it may also be used to treat oedema, cellulite, and any excess of fluid in the body. Its astringent action means it can be used to treat piles and prostatitis. As it eliminates waste it can be used to treat arthritis and other painful conditions of the joints, and here its warming action also helps. Skin conditions, including acne, ulcers, eczema, psoriasis, and dermatitis will also respond. It has an action on the digestive system, which means it can be used for loss of appetite, diabetes, and as a pancreatic stimulant to encourage a healthy appetite and good digestion. It will also act on excess mucus, both in chest infections and in the digestive system. As a sedative it can be used for insomnia, especially when it is caused by 'emotional toxicity'. However, as a physical stimulant it is useful for convalescence, since it calms the mind and tones the body. It has traditionally been used to clean the air and it does this on an emotional level as well. It is invaluable for clearing negative energies and is used by crystal healers to purify stones used for healing. If you are exposed to a negative influence or know that you are going to be, this oil will help. It is considered to protect the solar plexus.

**Cautions:** Avoid in kidney inflammation due to the diuretic actions. Probably best avoided during pregnancy.

## Lavandin (Lavandula x intermedia)

**Family:** Labiatae/Lamiacae

There are various different clones or strains of Lavandin, which is a hybrid between true Lavender and Spike Lavender. The clone which is most useful therapeutically is 'Super', since this is closest to true lavender. Others are Abrialis, Reyodan, and Grosso. It is best to buy this oil from an organic source. Clones are very vigorous and high yielding initially, but become weakened over generations. Uses similar to true lavender.

Obtained by steam distillation, mainly in France, but also in Spain, Hungary, Yugoslavia, and Argentina. The oil is colourless or pale yellow and has a camphorous odour when compared with true lavender (see below).

**Constituents:** Monoterpenes; limonene, cis and trans ocimenes. Alcohols; linalool, borneol. Esters; linalyl acetate, bornyl acetate, lavandulyl acetate, geranyl acetate. Ketones; camphor/borneol. Coumarins; coumarin, herniarin.

## Lavender (Lavandula officinalis, vera, angustifolia)

**Family:** Lamiacae/Labiatae

The plant is a perennial herb, growing up to three foot in height. It has silver/green lanceolate leaves and bears small typical lamiate flowers from mid-summer. These may be varying shades of blue/purple, although they are occasionally pink or white. The herb is still used by herbalists, and the whole herb has similar properties to the essential oil in this case.

The essential oil is obtained by steam distillation of the flowering heads. it is a clear colourless to pale-yellow liquid, with a floral herbal aroma. Low altitude oils are more camphorous in odour, high altitude oils contain more esters. An absolute is also extracted for the perfumery industry. A hydrosol is also available. Mainly produced in France, Italy, Spain, Tasmania, Turkey, and Bulgaria. On some price lists, one sees 'Lavender 40/42'. This refers to the content of linalyl acetate. The higher the quantity the higher the price. However, view this with suspicion as it is perfumery terminology and, therefore, the oil is probably not prepared for the aromatherapy market. The production of Lavender oil from France has dropped dramatically in recent years due to a fungal disease affecting the plants but similar volumes continue to be exported, which means some of what is sold as Lavender oil is not. By supporting small scale farmers and distillers and asking your supplier questions about provenance, you can continue to be guaranteed that it is the true oil of suitable quality that you are obtaining. You may also wish to consider switching to oil from other territories such as Bulgaria.

Several other members of the Lavender family produce oils; Lavandin—a hybrid, Spike Lavender, and *L. stoechas*.

**Constituents:** Aldehydes (2%); myrtenal, cuminal, citral, geranial, trans-hexanal. Esters (40–50%); linalyl acetate, lavandulyl acetate, terpenyl acetate, geranyl acetate. Ketones (4%); camphor, octanone, p-methyl-acetophenone. Oxides (2%); 1,8-cineole, linalol oxide, caryophyllene oxide. Monoterpenols; linalol, terpin-4-ol, $\alpha$-terpineol, borneol, geraniol, lavandulol. Coumarins/lactones; herianin, coumarin, umbelliferone, santonin.

**Actions:** Adrenal cortex stimulant, analgesic, anticoagulant, anticonvulsive, antidepressant, antifungal, antishock, antispasmodic, antiviral, bactericidal (diptheria and typhoid bacilli, streptococcus and pneumococcus), bechic, cardiac tonic, carminative, CNS regulator, cholagogue, choleretic, cicatrisant, cordial, cytophylactic, deodorant, emmenagogue, hypotensive, immuno-stimulant, insecticide, mucolytic, nervine, parasiticide, rubefacient, sedative, sudorific, tonic, vulnerary.

**Uses:** Lavender oil is regarded in the aromatherapy world as a real cure-all, and it does indeed have a multitude of application, as well as being very safe to use. It is one of the oils that can be used safely during delivery and on newborn infants. Lavender baths during labour have been reported to make the process shorter and smoother. On babies the oil can be used for a wide range of problems—it soothes colic and the pain of teething. Lavender is also sedative for the restless child and can be used for nappy rash, eczema, and other skin eruptions. In pregnancy, it may be inhaled for morning sickness and applied over the abdomen from the fifth month to help prevent stretch marks. It is an antifungal oil and is, therefore, used for athlete's foot, ringworm, and candida (thrush, rectal, oral, nail infections). It is used for abscesses, acne, boils, sores, spots, allergies, dermatitis, eczema, and psoriasis. As a skin regenerator, Lavender heals bruises and wounds, burns and sunburn, dandruff, earache, inflammations, insect bites and stings, and varicose ulcers. It is an insect repellent and parasiticide, which is active against flies, dust mites, lice and scabies, as well as moths.

As an analgesic, it is useful for muscular aches and pains, rheumatism, and arthritis. It is also used for headaches, migraine. Lavender is a nervous system regulator and is therefore sedative at lower doses, becoming stimulating at higher doses. Used for insomnia, anxiety, depression, PMS, menopausal mood disturbances, panic attacks, and shock. Lavender may also be used for the treatment of sinusitis, otitis, cystitis, herpes, pruritis, influenza, spasmodic coughs. Asthma, bronchitis, catarrh, and throat infections.

Lavander is a cardiotonic for tachycardia and palpitations, lowers blood pressure, and is used for menstrual pain, gastric cramps, and nausea. Blends well with most other oils, particularly the herbs, citrus and other florals. On the emotional and spiritual level, Lavender is used for its cleansing properties. It is reputed that it helps to balance the psyche.

**Cautions:** Although there have been some reports of skin irritation, they have not specified the use of an unadulterated oil, and since Lavender is widely adulterated, such reports may be inaccurate. The oil is generally regarded as an emmenagogue, and therefore it should be used in the first trimester of pregnancy. As a hypotensor the oil may cause extreme drowsiness in individuals with low blood pressure.

### Lemon (Citrus limomum per.)

**Family:** Rutaceae

In common with the other citrus trees, the Lemon is a small evergreen, bearing white flowers. It probably originated in India, but now grows throughout the Mediterranean. The main areas of production are Italy, Sicily, Cyprus, Israel, and the Americas. The true oil is produced by cold expression from the rinds. It is important to obtain an oil that is prepared from unsprayed fruit. However, a distilled oil is also produced for the food industry. The aroma of the distilled oil is closer to that of fresh lemons. The fresh oil is a bright yellow with a characteristic scent. Deterpenated oils are not suitable for use therapeutically due to the concentration of citrals that occurs in this process.

**Constituents:** Monoterpenes; limonene (<80%), pinenes, terpinene, sabinene, thujene, myrcene, phellandrene, terpinene, cymene. Sesquiterpenes; bisabolene, bergamotine, caryophyllene. Monoterpenols; linalol, terpineol-4, terpineol. Aldehydes; geranial, neral, citronellal, nonanal, octanal, decanal. Esters; neryl acetate, geranyl acetate, terpinyl acetate. Coumarins; bergamotine, citropen, bergaptol, phellopterin, bergaptene.

**Actions:** Anti-anaemic, antibacterial, anti-coagulant, alkaline form-
ing, anti-infectious, anti-inflammatory, antisclerotic, antiseptic, antispasmodic, antiviral, astringent, carminative, calming, deodoriser,
diuretic, digestive, depurative, febrifuge, fumigant, immune-modulant,
litholytic, pancreatic stimulant, phlebotonic, stomachic.

**Uses:** Lemon is valuable in the treatment of water retention, obesity,
and cellulite. It is also a circulatory tonic, normalising blood pressure
and helping to clear the arteries. It is particularly useful for strengthening the capillary circulation and is used for chilblains and for conditions of capillary fragility, such as thread veins, varicose veins, and
haemorrhoids. According to Penoel and Franchomme (1995), it is also
useful for the treatment of phlebitis and thromboses, but this may be
via the oral route. Lemon encourages the production of white blood
cells so is useful in the treatment of a compromised immune system.
It appears to encourage red blood cell production as well and therefore may be indicated for anaemia. Lemon can be used for spontane-
ous bleeding and internal haemorrhages as well as blood in the saliva
or urine.

As a liver decongestant, it helps with hangovers, digestive dysfunc-
tion, and hyperacidity. It is a pancreatic stimulant, which means it could
be helpful in diabetes and hyperglycaemia. Other actions on the digestive system mean that it can be used to treat diarrhoea and dysentery,
hyperacidity, nausea, flatulence, constipation, and slow digestion.

Due to the aldehydes, Lemon can be used as a treatment for kidney
stones and gallstones.

It is used for respiratory infections, where it helps clear excess mucus
and as a fumigant to purify the air. It's antibacterial action makes it
appropriate for use against boils, abscesses, otitis, streptococcal tonsilitis, gingivitis, bronchitis, bacterial pneumonia, and tuberculosis of
the lungs or bones. It is a febrifuge effective for fevers, influenza, and
malarial or typhus fevers. It can also help with cold sores, especially
when mixed with Bergamot, Tea Tree, and Eucalyptuses (prefer *E.
smithii* or *radiata*).

As Lemon helps to reduce acidity and clears toxins from the body,
it can be valuable in the treatment of arthritis, gout, and rheumatism.

In skin care Lemon can be used at low dilutions for sensitive skins.
It is useful for oily hair and skins and helps to revive a sagging com-
plexion, since it encourages the removal of dead cells. As an astringent

it is particularly useful in the treatment of overactive skin and in the treatment of acne. When using Lemon oil for the treatment of corns, verrucae, and warts, it can be applied neat or as a mixture with Tea Tree and Tagetes, with a cotton bud. The surrounding skin should be protected from the oil. When treating verrucae, cushion the area with non-medicated corn plasters or elephant felt since verrucae thrive on pressure and relieving the pressure will speed up treatment. The treatment can be dramatically successful, but it is necessary to apply the oil 2–3 times during the day. Soaking the nails in olive oil and lemon oil makes the less brittle. It may also be used against fungal skin infections, including ringworm, tinea, mange, and scabies.

For travellers in areas where the water is suspect, a drop of Lemon oil may be added to drinking water to purify it.

As a nerve restorative Lemon is used for fatigue, weakness, stress, and convalescence. It may also be helpful in palpitations. It has been shown to be particularly refreshing, giving an increased feeling of health and wellbeing. It is reputed to help clear and sharpen the mind, particularly useful for sharpening the concentration. It is also helpful for the begrudger who likes to bring others down and resents other's good fortune or success. It has a generally activating and stabilising action on the consciousness and is calming with a cooling, clearing, and refreshing action.

Gumbel (1984) says that the oil can encourage uterine contraction in an overdue delivery.

Any Lemon oil that is past its therapeutically useful life can be used to clean greasy marks from paint work and glass. It is an excellent cleaning agent for removing grease from the hands as well.

**Cautions:** In common with other monoterpene rich oils, Lemon should be used within a year of production. Keeping it refrigerated will cause the precipitation of non-volatile waxy constituents that are present in the expressed oil. It contains coumarins, including bergaptene, which means it can cause a phototoxic reaction if used before exposing the skin to UV radiation. It is not phototoxic below 10% dilution, since the percentage of furanocoumarins it contains is very low. The aldehydes it contains may give rise to skin irritation or sensitisation reactions in some individuals, therefore stick to low concentrations, except where specified. There are different opinions as to whether it should be used in pregnancy.

## Lemongrass (Cymbopogon spp.)

**Family:** Poaceae

### West Indian Lemongrass (Cymbopogon citratus)

West Indian Lemongrass is steam distilled from the fresh or partially dried grass. The oil is yellow to reddish brown. Native to Sri Lanka, but mainly cultivated in the West Indies, Africa, and Asia.

**Constituents:** Monoterpenes; limonene (1–11%). Monoterpenols; dipentene, linalol, geraniol, citronellol, farnesol. Aldehydes; neral (22–33%), geranial (37–45%), citronellal (1–13%).

**Cautions:** High concentrations may cause dermal irritation. Citral has also been shown to raise ocular tension which could cause problems for individuals with glaucoma.

### East Indian Lemongrass (Cymbopogon flexuosus)

The oil is yellow or amber. Mainly cultivated in western India.

**Constituents:** Monoterpenes; dipentene. Monoterpenols; geraniol, borneol, nerol, $\alpha$-terpineol. Sesquiterpenols; farnesol. Aldehydes (<85%); citrals. Phenyl methyl; ether methyl eugenol.

**Actions:** Similar in both species of Lemongrass. Analgesic, anti-inflammatory, antidepressant, antimicrobial, anti-oxidant, antiseptic, astringent, bactericidal, carminative, deodorant, febrifuge, fungicidal, galactogogue, insecticidal, nervine, sedative, tonic.

**Uses:** This oil is physically tonifying, yet balancing for the CNS. This means that its emotional effects, in regards to overstimulation or sedation depend on whether the individual is overstimulated and needs calming or under stimulated and needs to feel more alert. The herb has a long tradition of use in its native areas as an infusion taken to aid sleep and for digestive problems. The oil is used in skin care to treat fungal infections, particularly athlete's foot. Also used for excessive perspiration and as an insect repellent. It can also be used in a steam for open pores and to tighten and tone the skin. Its insecticidal properties can be used to treat lice and scabies. The oil can be used to stimulate the circulation and to treat muscular aches, particularly when due to overwork. It helps to improve the tone of the muscles and the tissues. As a carminative it may be used to treat digestive complaints, including colitis, indigestion, and gastroenteritis. It helps to regulate fever and therefore can be used for any febrile condition. As a sedative and CNS regulator it can be used to treat headaches, nervous exhaustion, and stress. Its anti-inflammatory properties can also be employed for the treatment of an inflammatory condition.

## Mandarin (Citrus reticulata per.)

**Family:** Rutaceae

Mandarin oil is expressed from the rinds of the fruit. The oil is a yellow/orange colour and has a slight fluorescence due to the presence of methyl anthranilate. This also gives the oil a slight fish odour! This oil is not to be confused with Tangerine, which does not contain methyl anthranilate and, therefore, is not as valuable therapeutically. The tree is a native of China and was highly prized, hence the name Mandarin. It is now grown in Italy, Spain, Cyprus, Brazil, and the Middle East.

**Constituents:** Monoterpenes; limonene, pinenes, myrcene, terpinene, terpinolene, cymene, phellandrene. Monoterpenols; citronellol, linalol, terpineol. Aldehydes; decanal, sinensal, perillaldehyde, octanal. Phenols; thymol. Esters; methyl anthranilate, benzyl acetate.

**Actions:** Antiepileptic, antifungal, antispasmodic, calming, carminative, cholagogue, digestive stimulant, mild diuretic, hepatic, mild hypnotic, lymphatic stimulant, stomachic, sedative, tonic.

**Uses:** Described as uplifting, but relaxing. It is an extremely safe oil, which can be used in pregnancy and on infants. Although it is very safe and gentle, it is very effective. I have found it invaluable for insomnia in children and also in stressed-out executives. In common with Orange, it is a nourishing oil with a particular affinity to the digestive system. It can help with loss of appetite and digestive problems, especially of nervous origin. It stimulates the liver and stomach, and therefore can be of benefit for flatulence and painful digestion. It helps with excesses of rich food and alcohol, and according to Patricia Davis (1988) can be useful for liver toxicity due to cannabis abuse. It is safe for sensitive skins and can be used for scars and the prevention of stretch marks. Congested and oily skins can also benefit. It may also be used for the treatment of water retention and cellulite and can be used for these during pregnancy. On an emotional level, I have found it to be an oil that nourishes the inner child. It has a definite affinity for the solar plexus, encouraging expansion and warmth in this area. Mandarin is generally regarded to balance the CNS and to be a gentle hypnotic.

**Cautions:** Non-toxic and non-irritant.

## Manuka (Leptospermum scoparium)

**Family:** Myrtaceae

It is steam distilled from the leaves of a New Zealand tree. The tree is also known locally as Tea tree, but is only distantly related to *Melaleuca alternifolia*, and therefore it's uses differ somewhat. The honey from forests of Manuka trees appears to have an action against the *Helicobacter pyrogenes* bacterium, which has been implicated in stomach ulcers.

**Constituents:** Monoterpenes; pinene, terpinene, myrcene, para-cymene, limonene Sesquiterpenes (65%); cubebene, yanglene, copaene, elemene, caryophyllene, selinene, aromadendrene, selinene, farnesene, calamanene, ∂-cadinene, cadina-1,4-diene, and others. Alcohols; spathulenol, cubenol. Oxides; caryophyllene epoxide. Ketones (25%); flavesone, isoleptospermone, leptospermone.

**Uses:** Has been shown to be even more affected against MRSA than *Melaleuca alternifolia*, and I would suggest that a synergistic blend of the two could be the best therapeutic option against this infection. The traditional uses of the plant include as an analgesic for muscular pain and rheumatism, as an insecticide, especially useful for keeping pets free of fleas. It has also been used for skin care in the treatment of boils, spots and other infected skin conditions. The ketones make it particularly valuable where there is slow healing. The ketones also make it valuable for the treatment of catarrhal conditions such as sinusitis, bronchitis and so on. Its analgesic action makes it useful for including in a gargle for sore throats too. It also appears to be effective against cold sores, although *Eucalyptus smithii/Eucalyptus globulus* are the most effective oils for treating these.

**Cautions:** Since this oil is high in ketones, it is only sensible to avoid its use in pregnancy. Ketones are potentially damaging to the foetus. It should also be used with caution on epileptics.

## Marjoram, Spanish (Thymus mastichina)

**Family:** Labiatae/Lamiacae

**Constituents:** Monoterpenes; terpinolene (4%), limonene (2–3%), ∂-pinene (2.6%), β-pinene (2–3%), para-cymene (1–3%), sabinene 1%, thujene, myrcene, camphene, terpinene. Sesquiterpenes; β-caryophyllene, gurjunene, aromadendrene, cadinenes, β-bourbonene, caryophyllene. Monoterpenols; borneol, linalol (43%), ∂-terpineol (8%), geraniol, thujanols, pinocarveol, terpineols. Phenols; thymol (0–5%). Ketones; camphor (0–4%). Oxides; 1,8-cineole (41–75%), caryophyllene oxide. Esters; linalyl acetate, terpinyl acetate, bornyl acetate, trans-pinocarveol acetate, terpinyl acetate, geranyl acetate trans-sabinene hydrate.

**Actions:** Anti-infectious, antibacterial.

**Uses:** Sinusitis, catarrhal bronchitis, viral and bronchial infections.

**Cautions:** Probably best avoided in pregnancy due to the presence of phenols and ketones.

## Marjoram, Sweet (Origanum marjorana)

**Family:** Labiatae/Lamiacae

Steam distilled from the flowering tops, the aroma of the oil can vary quite measurably, but the true Sweet Marjoram oil has a sweet aroma due to the linalol, whereas Spanish Marjoram has a camphorous odour due to the presence of large amounts of cineole. Oreganos have a phenolic smell. The oil is pale yellow to amber in colour. It is mainly produced in France (the best quality), Tunisia, Morocco, Egypt, Bulgaria, Hungary, and Germany.

**Constituents:** Monoterpenes (40%); sabinene (2–10%), myrcene (1–9%), para-cymene (1–6%), terpinolene (1–7%), pinene (1–5%), ß-pinene 0–3%, ocimene 6%, cadinene 4%, carene 6%, terpinene, phellandrene, myrcene, limonene. Sesquiterpenes: $\beta$-caryophyllene (2–5%), -humulene. Monoterpenols (50%); terpineol-4 (14–20%), thujanol-4s (5–15%), linalol (2–9.5%), -terpineol (7–27%), menthenol, piperitol. Esters; terpenyl acetate, geranyl acetate, linalyl acetate. Aldehydes; citral (5%).

**Actions:** Analgesic, anaphrodisiac, anti-infectious, antispasmodic (particularly gastric), antibacterial, calming, digestive stimulant, diuretic, emmenagogue, expectorant, thyroid regulator, hypotensive, nervine, respiratory tonic, rubefacient, sedative, vasodilator.

**Uses:** A particularly warming oil, both physically and emotionally. This makes it valuable for the treatment of muscular and joint pains, including arthritis and rheumatism, muscular spasms, cramps and fibrositis, especially as it has analgesic properties as well.

Its analgesic and nervine properties make it valuable for migraine, toothache, tics, and neurasthenia. A warm compress on the back of the neck can be very effective at warding off a migraine before it becomes full blown, partly due to the fact it dilates the blood vessels. Marjoram can also be helpful in the treatment of other forms of headache.

In common with other members of the Labiate family, Majoram is useful for treating digestive problems. It helps dispel flatulence, colic, and indigestion. It is also an excellent treatment for constipation when used with abdominal massage. However, it can also be used to treat diarrhoea, since it encourages a regular and smooth peristalsis. Because it is used for nervous conditions, it can also help relieve stress-related peptic ulcers. Also, its anti-infectious property makes it a treatment for enteritis.

As the oil is vasodilatory and calming, it lowers the blood pressure very effectively. In this instance, baths (not too hot!) and massage are particularly effective because they both will enhance this effect. This property also makes it useful for treating bruises and strains. It can also be used for the treatment of tachycardia and palpitations.

Because of the antispasmodic property, it is used for period pains and cramps. It will also help with bronchial spasm and I know of several asthmatics who find it particularly useful as a prophylactic when used in the burner. Staying with the respiratory system it can be used for whooping cough (preferably in a steam diffuser and/or steamy baths), bronchitis, rhinitis, sinusitis, catarrh, coughs, and respiratory infections.

Its effect on the mind and emotions Is also marked and makes it valuable in treating various 'nervous' conditions. It has been used by appropriately trained practitioners in the treatment of addictions, psychosis, and mental instability. However, in the average aromatherapy practice it is more likely to be used for extreme anxiety and hysteria, especially where insomnia or hyperpnoea are symptoms or for nervous depression. It can be very helpful in the acute stages of grief, allowing the individual to feel an emotional warmth and enabling them to cope with day to day. But do remember the caution about overuse. Also used for debility. Its anaphrodisiac property makes it an oil that can help with sexual obsessions or to be used for people going through a time of enforced celibacy, such as bereavement or the absence of a partner— also good for loneliness.

Other instances where it can be used include the treatment of vertigo and nervous tics. It can be used for people with epilepsy and seems to regulate overactivity in the thyroid gland.

**Cautions:** Avoid in pregnancy, but this may be due to confusion with phenol-rich origanums. Overuse can lead to numbing of the emotions, so stick to the rule of altering oils used every two to three weeks.

## May Chang, Exotic Verbena, Tropical Verbena (Litsea cubeba)

**Family:** Lauraceae

A small evergreen tropical tree, native to east Asia, especially China, but also cultivated in Taiwan and Japan. The oil is mainly produced in China, where the trees are grown as wind breaks. The leaves and flower smell similar to Lemongrass, due to their citral content. The fruits are shaped like peppers, hence the name *cubeba*. The oil is steam distilled from the fruits and is pale yellow. It is generally considered non-toxic and safe to use but may cause sensitisation of the skin in sensitive individuals. Should be used in low concentrations like all aldehyde-rich oils.

**Constituents:** Citral (up to 85%), linalol, linalyl acetate, cineole, cadinene, limonene, sabinene.

**Actions:** Antidepressant, antiseptic, deodorant, digestive, disinfectant, insecticidal, stimulant, stomachic, tonic, astringent.

**Uses:** Acne, dermatitis, greasy skin, flatulence, and indigestion. Can be a useful tonic, revitalising, low energy, and may be helpful for bronchitis and asthma. Sellar (1992) reports that it can be helpful for coronary heart disease.

## Melissa/Lemon Balm (Melissa officinalis)

**Family:** Lamiaceae

Steam distilled from the flowering tops, Melissa herb contains less than 0.01% of volatile oil, which is why it is so expensive. Mainly cultivated in France, Spain, Germany, and Russia. The only essential oil to be produced in Ireland.

**Constituents:** Monoterpenes; ocimene, bourbonene, limonene. Sesquiterpenes; β-caryophyllene (8–10%), germacrene, copaene (4–5%), elemene, humulene, cadinene. Monoterpenols; linalool, nerol, geraniol, citronellol, isopulegol. Sesquiterpenols; cadinol, elemol. Ketones; methylheptenone, hexahydrofarnysyl acetone. Esters; geranyl acetate, neryl acetate, citronellyl acetate. Oxides; 1,8-cineole, caryophyllene oxide. Aldehydes; neral (22–24%), geranial (32–37%), citronellal. Coumarin; aesculetine.

**Actions:** Anti-inflammatory, antispasmodic, calming, choleretic, digestive, hypotensor, sedative, vasodilator.

**Uses:** The choleretic action is very powerful—bile production is tripled within half an hour. This makes it valuable for poor or sluggish digestion. It can also be used to treat stomach cramps, indigestion, nausea, morning sickness, and a sluggish liver. The aldehydes also mean it is indicated for gallstones. It's calming action is excellent. It can be used for all types of insomnia and any nervous problems, such as depression, PMS, and menopausal mood swings. Davis (1991) cites it as chasing away the black spirits and it truly seems to lift the mood. Also good for hysteria, shock, palpitations, and vertigo. It is a hypotensor, which is invaluable in treating high blood pressure and may also relieve angina. The hydrosol can help to regulate fever, particularly in children, as can the tisane. It is also active against *Herpes simplex*, healing the lesions more quickly and lessening the frequency of recurrence. Low concentrations of the oil can be used in the treatment of skin allergies, such as eczema, but only under 1%. It is also indicated for asthma, bronchitis, and chronic coughs.

Davis (1991) says that it can help acceptance of death. Also, Lemon Balm has an affinity to the Heart chakra.

**Cautions:** Care may be necessary in sunlight. Also, low concentrations are preferable due to the high concentration of aldehydes in the oil, particularly when treating respiratory problems and skin allergies. Care to obtain the true oil, which is at least as expensive as rose, since it is frequently sold as an adulterated oil.

## Myrrh (Commiphora molmol/myrrha)

**Family:** Burseraceae

**Constituents:** Sesquiterpenes (39%); elemens, copaene. Ketones (6%); curzeronone, methyl isobutyl ketone. Aldehyde; methyl butenal.

**Actions:** Anticatarrhal, anti-inflammatory, antiseptic, astringent, emmenagogue, expectorant, fungicidal, stomachic, tonic, uterine, vulnerary. Possibly an anaphrodisiac.

**Uses:** The main actions are drying up excess moisture (sesquiterpenes) and healing. Its healing property can be used in the treatment of athlete's foot, gingivitis, mouth infections, mouth ulcers and pyorrhoea (although it tastes very bitter—tincture of myrrh can be used as an equally bitter alternative), haemorrhoids, throat infections, skin ulcers, weeping skin and wounds. I have seen it work in the treatment of a non-granulating area of skin from which grafting material was taken when nothing else would.

Due to its action on excess moisture, it can be used to treat catarrh in the respiratory system and bowel, as well as diarrhoea. Also cited for hyperthyroidism and thrush.

**Cautions:** Avoid during pregnancy due to uterine effect.

## Myrtle (Myrtus communis)

**Family:** Myrtaceae

Myrtle is a close relative of Eucalyptus and the aroma closely resembles this oil. It is, however, lighter and fresher, with an almost floral note. This makes it more tolerable for a lot of people.

There are various myrtle oils available, all from the same species— red, orange and green varieties are sold. These differ slightly in their stimulating/sedative quality, with the red oil being more stimulating and the orange oil being more sedative. The oil is steamed distilled from the leaves and varies in colour from pale yellow to a deep amber. There is also a hydrolat available which is traditionally used in skincare and is reputed to encourage the eyebrows to grow healthily!

**Constituents:** 1,8-cineole. Alcohols; myrtenol, geraniol, linalool. Monoterpenes; pinene, camphene.

**Actions:** Antiseptic, antibacterial, astringent, slightly sedative.

**Uses:** Chest infections and pulmonary catarrh. Because it is more sedative than some of the other cineole rich oils, it is valuable for using in a diffuser in the evening and through the night to help clear the chest. Urinary and vaginal infections. Also, may be used for acne and congested skin.

Red myrtle in morning, and orange myrtle at night.

**Cautions:** Generally considered to be a gentle oil which can be used safely on children, babies, and frail people.

## Neroli (Citrus aurantium ssp. aurantium flos)

**Family:** Rutaceae

The essential oil is obtained by steam distillation of the flowers of the bitter orange. Essential oil obtained from the sweet orange flowers is not ideal and is known as Portugal Neroli. Neroli bigarade is the desired article. The oil is pale yellow, darkening with age, and is a mobile liquid. An absolute is also extracted and is a brown/orange viscous liquid, but has a deep, almost nauseating aroma and is not suitable for use therapeutically. A hydrosol is also available and may be used in skin care. It is also used in Middle Eastern cookery. Main areas of production are Italy, Tunisia, Morocco, Egypt, America, and France.

**Constituents:** Monoterpenes (35%); $\alpha$-pinene, $\beta$-pinene (13%), limonene (12–18%). Alcohols; monoterpene $\alpha$-terpineol (5%), linalol (30%), geraniol (3%), nerol (3%). sesquiterpene nerolidol (6%), farnesol. Aromatic alcohols; phenyl ethyl alcohol, benzyl alcohol. Esters; linalyl acetate (5%), neryl acetate 3%, geranyl acetate (1%), methyl anthranilate. Aldehydes; nerals. Ketones; jasmone (non-toxic).

**Actions:** Anti-infectious, anti-parasitic, antidepressive, anti-tumour, antibacterial, digestive, neurotonic, sedative, hypotensive, phlebotonic, antispasmodic.

**Uses:** A digestive tonic due to its action on the liver and pancreas; may also be useful for diabetes. It is used for diarrhoea and digestive upsets, especially when nervous in origin, since it is also neurotonic. Combined with its antispasmodic action, it could be valuable in the treatment of IBS and spastic colon. It is an excellent tonic for the nervous system used for fatigue, insomnia, and depression. It is traditionally used for lack of confidence, and extreme nervous or anxious states, particularly stage fright and exam nerves. It may be useful for recovery from shock, although true shock is a severe trauma to the system and requires medical attention. It is an excellent tonic for the cardiovascular system, used for hypertension—especially arterial, varicose veins, and haemorrhoids—possibly for varicose ulcers also and all other varicosities, although there are many other oils which might be first preference here. The esters make it a powerful antispasmodic, including for uterine spasm since it is a uterine tonic. It is also quoted as being useful in bronchitis and pleurisy, possibly due to its antispasmodic action. It is cytophylactic, promoting the growth of healthy skin cells, making it valuable for dry and sensitive skins, and skin complaints of nervous origin. Due to its lack of toxicity, it may also be used throughout pregnancy to treat stretch marks. On an emotional level, it is valuable for extreme nervousness with anxiety and disturbance.

## Niaouli (Melaleuca quinquinervia/viridiflora)

**Family:** Myrtaceae

Niaouli contains more than 110 components! The oil is steam distilled from the young leaves and twigs. It is pale to dark yellow, almost brown on occasion. It is produced in Madagascar, Australia and New Caledonia. Sometimes called Gomenol.

**Constituents:** Monoterpenes; pinenes, phellandrene, terpinenes, limonene. Sesquiterpenes; β-caryophyllene, aromadendrenes, viridiflorene, cadinene. Monoterpenols; linalol, terpineol-4. Sesquiterpenols; globulol, viridiflorol, nerolidol. Oxides; 1,8-cineole. esters and aldehydes maybe also be present.

**Actions:** Anti-allergic, antibacterial, anti-infectious, anti-inflammatory, anti-parasitic, antiseptic, antiviral, balsamic, expectorant, hepatic tonic, hormone-like, hypotensive, litholytic, phlebotonic and decongestant, radio-protective.

**Uses:** As a cardiac tonic it can be used for hypertension, atherosclerosis, and endocarditis. It is also indicated for haemorrhoids and varicosities. It is excellent for the treatment of chronic respiratory catarrh, for instance chronic bronchitis, sinusitis, or pharyngitis. It can be used for a wide range of vaginal infections, where it's hormonal action also helps—herpes, leucorrhoea, and Thrush. It is used for a range of gastrointestinal problems, including viral hepatitis, gastritis, aerophagy, gastric and duodenal ulcers, and viral enteritis. As a liver tonic, it can ease gallstones and help strengthen the liver during convalescence or when it is weakened by stress. In the urinary system it can be used for prostatitis and urethritis. for skin care it is indicated for psoriasis of all types, acne (especially when hormone related), and fungal dermatitis. It can also help in hormone related arthritis and rheumatism. Niaouli is a boost to the nervous system and can help with depression and nervous exhaustion, being a stimulant. A thin layer of Niaouli oil can help to prevent radiation burns, or at least lessen their severity.

**Cautions:** Use sparingly in pregnancy and with young children.

## Nutmeg (Myristica fragrans)

**Family:** Myristicaceae

Obtained by steam distillation from the Nutmeg seed, normally worm eaten to remove the fats and starches. An oil is also obtained from the 'mace', which surrounds the kernel, but this is rare.

**Constituents:** Monoterpenes (70–75%); pinene, myrcene, sabinene, terpinene, limonene, phellandrene, camphene, cymene, terpinolene. Sesquiterpenes; β-caryophyllene. Monoterpenols; terpineol-4, α-terpineol, linalol, geraniol, borneol. Phenyl ethers (4%); safrole, myristicin, elemi-cin, eugenol, methyl eugenol. Oxides; 1,8-cineole.

**Actions:** Analgesic, antibacterial, antiseptic, carminative, circulatory stimulant, digestive stimulant, emmenagogue, tonic, uterine, nervine.

**Uses:** As an analgesic used to treat rheumatism, muscular aches and pains, sprains, toothache, and neuralgia. As a carminative used for chronic diarrhoea, gallstones, loss of appetite, and sluggish digestion, especially where starches cause problems. As regards the reproductive system, it is used for scanty periods, frigidity, and impotence and can facilitate delivery.

Also used for chills, due to its warming effect. It has also been used in embalming to preserve corpses.

**Cautions:** Prolonged use can irritate the skin. Avoid in pregnancy. Large doses stimulate the cerebral cortex and may cause epileptic like seizures. The whole spice is narcotic in large amounts, but this does not apply to the oil.

## Orange, Bitter (Citrus aurantium ssp. Aurantium per.)

**Family:** Rutaceae

Sweet Orange (*Citrus sinensis per.*) Is similar to bitter orange, but with no phototoxic effect. According to one source (Clifford, per. Comm.), it is more appropriate for physical ailments, whilst Bitter Orange has a greater affinity for the emotions and for solar plexus work. According to Gumbel (1984), Sweet Orange oil will raise blood sugar levels. He describes the oil as promoting warmth.

**Constituents:** Monoterpenes; limonene, myrcene, terpinolene, pinene, camphene.

Sesquiterpenes; caryophyllene, copaenes, farnesene, humulene. Alcohols; citronellol, terpineol, nerol, linalol, nerol, geraniol. Alde-hydes; geranial, neral, undecanal, sinensal. Esters; linalyl acetate, gera-nyl acetate, neryl acetate, citronellyl acetate. Coumarins; trace.

**Actions:** Antidepressant, anti-inflammatory, antiseptic, calming, carminative, cholagogue, digestive, hypotensive, sedative, stomachic, tonic, stimulant to the digestive and lymphatic systems.

**Uses:** Orange has been described as a nourishing oil. It can be helpful for people who are feeling emotionally low, especially when this affects their digestion and appetite. It is a sedative antidepressant oil, useful for insomnia and for low emotional states, especially when associated with coldness on a physical level, as it seems to have an affinity for the circulation. It's action on the pancreas and liver help with the digestive system in general. It can be used for gastric spasm and constipation. As a sedative it is useful for anxiety and nervousness, and it regulates the Central Nervous System. It may also be indicated in vertigo and palpitations. Price mentions it as being valuable in the treatment of gum infections and mouth ulcers, where its flavour may be more palatable than some of the other oils mentioned for these conditions.

**Cautions:** Phototoxicity with the expressed oil. Not recommended in pregnancy, since it may affect the foetus liver or on small infants as the liver cannot metabolise the oil until developed fully.

## Oregano (Origanum vulgare)

**Family:** Lamiaceae
**Constituents:** Terpinenes; thujene, pinenes. Myrcene; limonene, linalool, terpien-4-ol, borneol, thujan-4-ol, carvacrol, thymol, linalyl acetate, 1,8-cineole, carvone.
**Actions:** anti-infectious, antiparasitic, immunomodulant, antioxidant, tonic.
**Uses:** Treats a wide range of infections of the digestive respiratory and genitourinary systems. An energising tonic used to treat asthenia.

## Palmarosa (Cymbopogon martinii)

**Family:** Poaceae/Graminaceae
The oil is steam or water distilled from a tropical grass. It comes originally from India and Pakistan, but is now grown in Africa, Indonesia, Brazil, and the Comores. Due to its high content of geraniol, it was often used to adulterate rose oil. The oil is pale yellow to green and slightly viscous. Its aroma is very sweet due to the esters.
**Constituents:** Monoterpenols (80–95%); linalol, geraniol (80%), nerol, p-menthadienol. Sesquiterpenols; elemol. Esters; geranyl formiate, neryl formiate, geranyl acetate, p-menthadienol acetate, geranyl butyrate, prenyl isovalerate, geranyl isovalerate, amyl, prenyl and geranyl hexanoates, prenyl and geranyl octanoates.
**Actions:** Antiseptic, anti-fungal, antiviral, bactericidal, cicatrisant, digestive, febrifuge, hydrating, stimulant for the circulatory, nervous, reproductive, and digestive systems, tonic.

**Uses:** As an anti-infectious agent the oil can be used for upper respiratory tract infections, although it would not be a first choice. However, it is very useful for genito-urinary infections including cystitis, vaginitis, urethritis, thrush, and for delivery. It may also be used for bacterial and viral enteritis. The other area of use where it comes to the fore is in skin care. It is very effective for staphylococcal acne, where its nervous action is useful for the lack of confidence that also tends to accompany this condition. It may also be used for dry forms of eczema and dry skin due to age or stress, with attention to diet and lifestyle as well, and since it balances the sebum production it is valuable for all skin types. Also, scars, sores, and minor skin infections. As a circulatory tonic it can be used for cardiac fatigue. It's action on the nervous system makes it a valuable oil to use for conditions of a nervous origin. It has been used in the treatment of anorexia. It may also be indicated in digestive atonia—a particularly unpleasant stress-related condition where the digestive process breaks down, causing diarrhoea, vomiting, and malabsorption—again, a complex condition to treat. It is generally indicated for nervous exhaustion and stress-related problems. On the more subtle level, it would be regarded as having an affinity with the heart chakra, due to its pale green colour and 'pink' aroma. It is regarded as a useful healing oil for the spirit.

**Cautions:** Due to its high geraniol content some caution should be observed as regards long term use. It is generally considered to be non-toxic, and non-irritating.

## Patchouli (Pogostemon patchouli/cablin)

**Family:** Labiatae/Lamiacae

Distilled from the fermented leaves of a tropical relative of Mint, check for hints of minty odour. Produced in India, China, Malaysia, and South America. Patchouli is also distilled in Europe and USA from the dried leaves. Traditionally used in India to preserve cloth from insect attack.

**Constituents:** Monoterpenes; pinenes, limonene. Sesquiterpenes (40–50%); bulnesene, guaiene, patchoulene, seychellene, β-caryophyllene, cadinene, aromadendrene. Sesquiterpenols (35–45%); patchoulol, pogostol, bulnesol, guaiol. Ketones (1–3%) patchoulenones. Oxides; guaiene oxide, bulnesene oxide, caryophyllene oxide.

**Actions:** Anti-infectious, anti-inflammatory, antifungal, antiseptic, decongestant, cicatrisant, immuno-stimulant, insect repellent, phlebotonic.

**Uses:** Patchouli is an excellent oil for treating damp skin conditions and for skin care generally. Used for acne, inflamed skin, allergies, seborrhoeic eczema, cracked skin, scars, haemorrhoids, varicose veins. Also used for lowered immunity and enteritis. Another oil to use for oedema, water retention, and cellulite. Small amounts seem to sedate and larger amounts stimulate. It has a deep earthy smell and is considered to strengthen the base chakra. It also balances the sacral chakra and, therefore, helps with water balance. An oil that helps to earth us and put us in touch with our physical needs.

**Cautions:** None known. However, some people detest the aroma so check whether it is acceptable to the individual before using!

## Peppermint (Mentha x piperita)

**Family:** Lamiacae

Thought by some botanists to be a cross between *Mentha spicata* and *Mentha aquatica*. However, there is some disagreement about this. The best variety is 'Mitcham', which was developed in this part of England. However, the crop is no longer grown there but there is now a company distilling 'Mitcham' Peppermint in England again. Distilled from dried leaves which may be stored for up to three years before processing. The best quality oil is produced from the fresh flowering tops. The whole oil is more effective than the extracted menthol. Produced mainly in France, England, USA, Russia, Bulgaria, Italy, Hungary, Morocco, and China.

**Constituents:** Monoterpenes (3–18%); pinenes, limonene, menthene, phellandrene, sabinene, myrcene, ocimene, para cymene, terpinolenes, terpinenes. Sesquiterpenes; $\beta$-caryophyllene, farnesene, muurolene, germacrene, cadinene, bourbonene. Monoterpenols (50%); menthol (28–45%), piperitol, piperitenol, terpineol, linalool, terpineol-4. Sesquiterpenols. Ketones; menthone (16–36%), piperitone, pulegone (<1%). Oxides; 1,8-cineole. Esters; methyl acetate (1–10%), menthofuran.

**Actions:** Analgesic, antifungal, anti-infectious, anti-inflammatory, anti-lactogenic, antispasmodic, antiviral, antibacterial, carminative, cephalic, cordial, decongestant, digestive stimulant, expectorant, hepatic, hormonal, hypertensor, febrifuge, insect repellent, reproductive stimulant, stimulant, mucolytic, nervine, vasoconstrictor.

**Uses:** Perhaps best known for its action on the digestive system, hence after dinner mints etc. It's action on the liver and antispasmodic action make it a valuable digestive oil. It is still used in conventional medicine to treat irritable bowel syndrome in the form of capsules and can be used by aromatherapists applied over the abdomen for this purpose. Peppermint is used for diarrhoea, nausea, and vomiting, especially of a nervous origin. It's action on the liver makes it helpful in viral hepatitis, cirrhosis, and jaundice. It is also indicated for painful digestion, nausea, including travel sickness, gastritis, enteritis, indigestion, colitis, flatulence, gastric spasm, and colic. It's action on the digestion system is also one of the reasons it is excellent in the treatment of migraine.

The content of ketones makes it an excellent mucolytic, especially as an inhalant for sinusitis. Peppermint is also used for laryngitis, bronchitis, and bronchial asthma. However, in the last instance it should be used cautiously, as some asthmatics are allergic to the oil and find it induces spasm. Menthol causes cooling and increases blood supply to area where it is applied. It can therefore be used as a local refrigerant and analgesic for burns, knocks, inflamed skin, neuralgia, and sciatica. The cooling effect also helps reduce fever, but perhaps peppermint tea is this best way of using the herb in this instance—a blend of peppermint, elderflower, and yarrow herbs is particularly effective.

One area of application of peppermint that is often overlooked is its effect on the reproductive system. It stimulates the ovaries and therefore can help regulate infrequent periods. It may also help with impotence, although direct application would not be a sensible idea! It may also help ease childbirth and helps to dry up the flow of milk when weaning. In skin care, it can be used to treat ringworm and skin infections. Peppermint is also used for eczema, urticaria, herpes, skin irritation, redness, and rashes. However, do remember that it should not be applied over large areas and should only be used in low concentrations. It is an effective repellent for all sorts of undesirables, including gnats, mosquitoes, head lice, and scabies—as well as ants and rats.

Although not contraindicated in high blood pressure, Peppermint may help with low blood pressure. It can also be used to treat cystitis. On an emotional level, peppermint is well known for its cephalic properties—it helps clear the mind and clarify thinking processes. A useful oil for revising and studying. It also can help with apathy, nervous palpitations, and vertigo. Its action in the last condition is since it excites the motor nerves but dampens sensory nerves. Peppermint is a valuable oil to add to blends in tiny amounts to act as a catalyst and encourage penetration of the skin. Price (2007) recommends combining it with Ravensara (*Ravensara aromatica*) for analgesia. Do remember only to use on small areas and in low concentrations. Davis (1991) says that Peppermint helps to dispel pride and to overcome feelings of inferiority.

**Cautions:** Some individuals react to menthol with dermatitis, flushing, and headache, due to allergy. Avoid dermal application in pregnancy and infants under three years old. Low dilutions for skin irritation, do not use with homeopathy. The whole plant is more antispasmodic than menthol alone.

## Petitgrain (Citrus aurantium ssp. aurantium fol.)

**Family:** Rutaceae

**Constituents:** Monoterpenes (10%); myrcene, cymene, pinene, sabinene, phellandrene, sabinene, limonene. Alcohols; linalol, terpineol, nerol, geraniol, terpine-1ol-4, citronellol. Esters; linalyl acetate, neryl acetate, geranyl acetate, terpinyl acetate. Aldehydes; decanal, neral, geranial. Coumarins; citroptene, bergaptene.

**Actions:** The actions of Petitgrain are essentially very similar to those of Neroli. However, it is considered to have an inferior aroma and to be weaker in its action, particularly as a sedative and antispasmodic. Although this may be the case it is far more affordable and still has a place in practice.

## Pine (Pinus sylvestris)

**Family:** Pinaceae/Abiecaceae

Distilled from the needles and commonly adulterated with other conifers. Turpentine (the real stuff) is also distilled from various species and is used commonly as an adulterant of other essential oils, but has therapeutic properties of its own. The oil is pale yellow. Mainly from U.S.A., Russia, Scandinavia and Austria. The kernels are eaten as a restorative.

**Constituents:** Monoterpenes (60–70%); pinenes, limonene, carene, β-caryophyllene, camphene, sabinene, terpinene, ocimene, phellandrene, cymene, terpinolene. Sesquiterpenes; longifolene, cadinene, copaene. Monoterpenols; borneol, terpineol-4. Sesquiterpenols; cadinol, muurolol. Aldehydes; citronellal. Esters (1–10%); bornyl acetate.

**Actions:** Adrenal cortex stimulant, analgesic, anti-inflammatory, antifungal, anti-sudorific, antiseptic, bactericide, expectorant, insecticide, rubefacient, tonic (hormonal, pancreatic), vermifuge.

**Uses:** Although some people find the aroma rather too reminiscent of disinfectant, this oil is very valuable in practice. If the aroma is a deterrent, consider using one of the closely related species mentioned below.

Pine has always been associated with the respiratory system. The reason why sanatoriums for consumptives were built in the Alps was to allow the patients to benefit from the resins permeating the air, and the negative ions exuded by the trees. Sleeping in a Pine forest is also reputed to lengthen one's life. In practice, this affinity to the respiratory system may be valuable in the treatment of bronchitis, catarrh, colds, coughs, sinusitis, tracheitis, flu, and pneumonia. Pine has also been used in the treatment of tuberculosis. In addition, it can be useful in the treatment of asthma. It is especially valuable for the treatment of asthmatics who have been on long-term steroid treatment, since this can cause adrenal insufficiency and Pine can help to support the adrenal glands. Its antiseptic qualities are also used to treat cystitis, pyelitis, and other urinary infections. It is also used for prostatitis, ovarian congestion, impotence, and uterine problems. It has an analgesic action, which can be used to treat gout, arthritis, rheumatism, and muscular aches and pains. It has a deodorant property, which can be applied locally to sweaty feet (it also antiperspirant) or used to clean the air. It can be used in the treatment of lice, scabies, and in veterinary care.

Pine's action on the digestive tract indicates its use for gastralgia, intestinal pains, gallstones, other gall bladder problems, and for diabetes. Its tonifying action is indicated for hypotension, lymphatic congestion, debility, fatigue, and multiple sclerosis. Lastly, it may be used in the treatment of certain allergies and inflammations.

When combined with oxide-rich oils at a ratio of 1:5 it will help the speedy expectoration of catarrh and will help to dry up mucus. It can, therefore, be useful in severe infections accompanied by copious mucus production.

**Cautions:** Prolonged use, high concentrations on the skin, especially if prone to allergic reactions. All terpene-rich oils should be used within a year since they are very prone to oxidation. It is also important that the oil be correctly distilled since incorrect distillation may lead to the formation of breakdown products, which can cause dermal irritation and worsen allergic symptoms.

## Ravensara (Ravensara aromatica)

**Family:** Lauraceae

**Constituents:** Monoterpenes; pinenes, sabinene (13–15%). Sesqui-terpenes; β–caryophyllene. Monoterpenols; α-terpineol (6–7%), terpin-eol-4 (2%). Esters; terpenyl acetate. Oxides; 1,8-cineole (61%).

**Actions:** Anti-infectious, anti-inflammatory, antifungal, antiviral, antibacterial, expectorant, nervine.

**Uses:** This is an exceptionally useful oil for treating the immune system, for energising and for treating certain viral infections. It's anti-infectious and anti-inflammatory actions make it helpful in infections of the respiratory system, including rhinopharyngitis, flu, sinusitis, and bronchitis. It can also be used to treat whooping cough. For the digestive system, it can be used in the treatment of viral hepatitis and viral enteritis. The same would be true for the treatment of cholera. It's action on herpes, shingles and opthalmic shingles is truly spectacular. A graduate of mine used this oil for opthalmic shingles on a member of her family and the reduction in pain and vesiculisation was remarkable withing twenty-four hours. Also used for chicken pox and glandular fever. As regards its nervine action, it can be used to treat neuromuscu-lar complaints, insomnia, muscular fatigue, and seems to be energising. This last action makes it useful for people who are feeling debilitated and run down. Ravensara is very well-tolerated on the skin and there-fore can be applied neat to shingles and other skin conditions. Alterna-tively, a talc can be made from white clay to apply to chicken pox etc. It combines well with *Pelargonium graveolens* in the treatment of shingles and herpes. When massaged over the vertebral column gives relaxation according to Price and Price (2007).

**Cautions:** None known at usual doses. Very well tolerated even by sensitive skins. *Ravensara anisata* is an oil that needs to be used with caution. However, its aroma is very different and the two oils should not be easily confused.

## Rose (Rosa damascena/centifolia/gallica)

**Family:** Rosaceae

It may take a hundred kilos of petals to produce a few grams of the otto. There are thousands of species of rose, but the ones above are the ones used medicinally and to produce an essential oil. The oil is mainly produced in Morocco, Bulgaria, Turkey, and France. An absolute and concrete are also produced by solvent extraction. Whilst these have beautiful aromas and are cheaper, they are not suitable for use in clinical practice, although they may be used to make perfumes. The oil is a pale yellow and is quite viscous, occasionally becoming solid if the room temperature is low. This can usually be remedied by gently warming the bottle between the hands—do not heat by placing on a radiator or in boiling water. The absolute is a deep red/orange colour and is slightly less viscous and less prone to crystallisation. The Rose is a plant with huge mythology attached to it and appeals equally to men and women in fragrances. A phytol is also produced.

**Constituents:** Rose contains over 300 constituents. Monoterpenes; stearoptene (16%), pinenes, terpinene, limonene, myrcene, ocimene, para cymene, camphene, $\beta$-caryophyllene. Sesquiterpenes; octadecane, nonadecane, nonadecene. Monoterpenols; geraniol (15%), citronellol (22%), nerol (9%), linalol, iso-borneol, $\partial$-terpineol. Sesquiterpenols: farnesol, phenyl ethyl alcohol. Aldehydes; neral. Esters; citronellyl acetate, geranial, and neryl acetates. Phenyl methyl ethers; methyl eugenol. Oxides; rose oxides Others; damescenone, eicosane, heneicosane, docosane, tricosane, tetracosane, pentacosane.

The distilled oil is known as the otto and is produced from the petals of the rose. Despite the flowers being highly fragrant the yield is low, due to the delicacy of the molecules. Indeed, it is only due to developments in distillation technology that the distilled oil is vaguely affordable!

**Actions:** Antibacterial, anti-depressant anti-infectious, anti-inflammatory, antiseptic, antispasmodic, astringent, choleretic, cicatrisant, haemostatic, hepatic, laxative, sedative, splenetic, stomachic, nervine, uterine tonic, styptic.

**Uses:** Despite its high cost, Rose is an invaluable oil in practice. Bear in mind that its action is strong and therefore low dilutions can have marked effects. When you calculate the actual cost of the amount used in a treatment it is not that high. Some therapists charge more for creams or other preparations containing the oil after informing their clients. Its primary actions are as an antidepressant, reproductive tonic, and in skin care. In the reproductive area, it has many applications, which is interesting given that it is supposed to be governed by Venus. It is used to regulate the cycle, especially when disrupted by stress. It will also help reduce heavy periods. It may also increase fertility in men as well by raising the sperm count. It helps strengthen the uterine muscles and is therefore valuable used in the week before the due date and after delivery to return the uterus to normal quickly. As an antidepressant, it can also help to prevent the onset of post-natal depression, in conjunction with adequate nutrition. It can also be indicated in PMS and menopausal mood swings. It also has a reputation as an aphrodisiac.

These effects are not due to a direct hormonal action, but by acting as a tonic. It can also be used for depression and is invaluable for people who are grieving, which is interesting as it is supposed to be the aroma of sanctity. As an antidepressant it may be useful in the treatment of asthma, hay fever, and other stress-related conditions, as well as general debility, insomnia, and impotence. It acts both as a general tonic and as a neurotonic. In the area of skin care it can be used to help dry skin retain moisture and heal. The otto is very useful for dry, sensitive, and blotchy skins, but the absolute should not be used in this way. It can also be used to heal thread veins and broken capillaries. Rose is also useful to help prevent wrinkles, especially when combined with rosehip fixed oil. Eczema and psoriasis may also respond to the oil, and here it's action on the liver may come into action. As a cicatrisant and antiseptic, it may be used to treat mouth ulcers, gingivitis (taste may not appeal to everyone and there are plenty of other alternatives), and wounds—may be used for skin infections. The hydrolat is also used for the treatment of conjunctivitis. It's antiseptic action also makes it valuable for acute and chronic bronchitis. It is a circulatory tonic and can help with poor circulation. Rose is also a valuable tonic for the liver, useful for the treatment of recovering alcoholics. It has mild laxative actions and can be useful for nausea and stress-related digestive problems. On an energetic level, Rose has the reputation for strengthening both the two lowest chakras and the crown. It has an obvious affinity for the heart chakra, being linked with love, both physical and spiritual. It can be used for those whose heart has closed up due to grief. It is also excellent for those who have lost touch with their femininity, both male and female. Also helpful for linking the sacral and crown chakras and, therefore, may be helpful for those who feel guilty about physical intimacy. The herb is used for treating wounds and damaged skin. Its astringent actions are used in tonics for the digestive system and as a mild laxative.

**Cautions:** The absolute should not be used in high concentrations on the skin, due to the possibility of irritation by trace residues. The essential oil is non-toxic and non-irritant. Some authors suggest that it is avoided during early pregnancy, since it is a uterine tonic. Avoid in hypertension, or at least use sparingly.

### Rosemary (Rosmarinus officinalis/Salvia rosmarinus)

**Family:** Labiatae/Lamiacae

There are three different chemotypes of Rosemary. The race is similar in actions to the cineole/borneone types, and they are fairly similar in action to each other—although, the borneone/camphor type is the best general stimulant and for increasing energy, whilst the cineole type excels as a pulmonary decongestant and facilitates elimination from the liver and kidneys. The verbenone type differs somewhat, it strengthens the liver and gall bladder and is an excellent skin regenerator being gentle and non-irritant, and will be considered separately.

In general, the oil is extracted by steam distillation. The best quality oil comes from the flowering tops, whilst an inferior oil is extracted from the whole herb. A hydrolat is also available. The shrub is familiar to most people, and the leaves or branches can be used to make a tea and added to the bath. As well as the common Rosemary there are many cultivars, such as the Pine scented *R. officinalis var. angustifolius* and varieties with white or pink flowers, instead of the usual blue/ mauve flowers. Originally from the Mediterranean, the plant is now cultivated all over the world, but the main regions for oil production are France, Spain, and Tunisia. The oil is fluid and is colourless to pale yellow.

#### Wild Race/Cineole chemotype

**Constituents:** Monoterpenes; pinenes, camphene. Sesquiterpenes; $\beta$-caryophyllene. Esters; bornyl acetate. Oxides; 1,8-cineole. Ketones; borneone.

#### Borneone chemotype

Monoterpenes (39%); pinenes, camphene, myrcene, phellandrenes, limonene, terpinenes, para cymene. Sesquiterpenes;

β-caryophyllene (3%). Monoterpenols; linalool, terpineol-4, ∂-terpineol, borneol, thujanol-4, cymenol. Esters; bornyl acetate, fenchyl acetate. Oxides; 1,8-cineole (30%), caryophyllene oxide, humulene epoxide. Ketones; 3-hexanone, methylheptenone, borneone (30%), verbenone, carvone.

**Actions:** Analgesic, antimicrobial, antioxidant, antiseptic, antispasmodic, astringent, carminative, cephalic, cholagogue, choleretic, cicatrisant, cordial, cytophylactic, diaphoretic, digestive, emmenagogue, fungicidal, hepatic, hypertensive, nervine, parasiticide, restorative, rubefacient, stimulant (circulatory, adrenal cortex, and hepatic), stomachic, sudorific, vulnerary. Possible emmenagogue and diuretic.

**Uses:** Rosemary is well known for its stimulating effect on both the body and mind (Rosemary for remembrance). However, it's effects are far more far reaching than this.

It is a useful oil for digestive problems, due to its action on the liver and astringent actions. These mean that it can help both cholecystitis and gallstones (also hangovers!) It can also help diarrhoea, colitis, dyspepsia, flatulence, and liverish headaches, as well as the elimination of toxins from the system, including high levels of cholesterol. This makes it valuable for rheumatism and arthritis, especially with its adrenal cortex action. This may also be why some authors cite it as an emmenagogue.

Rosemary's high content of ketones and cineole together make it a valuable respiratory oil. It is indicated for colds, bronchitis, and flu. Also, for sinusitis, otitis, and other catarrhal conditions. It also seems to boost the immune system. The cineole type is effective against staphyloccocal, streptococcal, and *E. coli* infections, as well as klebsiella, proteus, and candida. The stimulating and rubefacient actions make it an oil that should be used at low concentrations in the bath and massage blends. However, it is an oil that is reputed to restore dulled senses, including sight and smell. I have seen it work to restore the sense of smell to individuals and there are many records of it being a valuable oil for elderly people. If the oil seems too strong, then the hydrolat can be used in foot baths. Rosemary also seems to help restore impaired nerve function, and is helpful for stress, mental fatigue, nervous exhaustion, and neuralgia. The oil is traditionally used to improve muscle tone and for reducing hypertonia in muscles, very useful for gardeners and sports people. Here, Rosemary is analgesic and rubefacient actions come into play and also make it valuable for period pains. As a circulatory tonic it is excellent for poor circulation, especially used in foot baths; also, for low blood pressure and varicose veins. Rosemary is valuable for the treatment of congested or overactive skin, dandruff, and oily hair. It is traditionally used on dark hair to keep the colour vibrant and is supposed to encourage healthy hair growth. The ketones make it useful for the treatment of burns. It can be helpful for getting rid of unwelcome guests, such as scabies and lice. Although normally cited as a stimulant that should not be used at night, I know of several people who find it sends them to sleep.

**Verbenone type**

**Constituents:** Monoterpenes ∂-pinene (15–34%); β-pinene, camphene, myrcene, limonene, terpinene, terpinolene. Sesquiterpenes; β-caryophyllene. Monoterpenols; borneol. Esters; bornyl acetate. Ketones; verbenone (15–37%), borneone (1–15%). Oxides; 1,8-cineole (20%).

**Actions:** Anticatarrhal, anti-infectious, antispasmodic, bactericide, cicatrisant, viricide, endocrine balancing, expectorant, mucolytic.

**Uses:** Used for sinusitis and bronchitis. As a tonic for the liver and gall bladder, therefore useful convalescent oil. May help diabetes. Used for leucorrhoea and regulating the reproductive hormones. It is especially useful for balancing the solar plexus and treating digestive problems of a nervous origin. Also, for nervous exhaustion, lowered libido, and depression. As a skin healer, it is excellent and may be used for scars, burns, acne, and dermatitis I have used it on psoriasis and eczema with good results.

**Cautions:** Due to the ketone content, Rosemary is normally considered best avoided during pregnancy, and also for people with epilepsy. It is also contraindicated for hypertensive individuals.

## Sandalwood (Santalum album)

**Family:** Santalaceae

The best quality oil comes from the Mysore region of India and is usually labelled "Agmark", a sign of good quality. Several other species are called Sandalwood, but do not have the same actions, so make sure you are getting the real thing—it is more expensive, as usual. The oil is steam distilled from the heart wood of the tree. Traditionally the timber is left to be attacked by termites, who eat off the outer layers, but leave the aromatic heart wood. This insect repellent quality is the reason why Sandalwood timber is widely used to make furniture in the tropics.

The oil contains a constituent that is similar to a human pheromone—aldosterone, which may explain its aphrodisiac reputation. An oil with huge mythology and traditional use attached to it. One should also consider that the production of this oil can have an environmental impact so should be used sparingly.

**Constituents:** Sesquiterpenes; santalenes, curcumenes, farnesene. Sesquiterpenols (>60%); santalols, lanceol, nuciferol. Aldehydes; teresantalal.

**Actions:** Anti-infectious, antispasmodic, astringent, carminative, cardiotonic, diuretic, expectorant, hydrating, nervine, tonic.

**Uses:** An extremely safe oil, which can be used in pregnancy without any worries. It's main areas of application are as an anti-infectious agent and in skin care. It can be used for infections of the respiratory system, urinary tract, reproductive organs, and skin. Being sedative, it is a useful oil to use for dry coughs at night. As a chest application it can help to relieve chronic bronchitis, and catarrh. For cystitis and other urinary infections, it is both soothing and anti-infectious, used for a local wash or douching. Sandalwood can also be used in an application cream. It has been shown to be effective against gonorrhoea and it may help with congested conditions of the pelvis and with diarrhoea. It also has a reputation for helping in the treatment of impotence and frigidity. In treating the skin, it can be used in massage, creams, or compresses, to treat all dry skin conditions. Sandalwood also helps regulate the production of sebum and therefore can also be used for oily skin and conditions that may respond include acne and eczema. Its antidepressant action is more appropriate for tension, anxiety, and insomnia caused by depression. This is because it calms the CNS. It has a phlebotonic action, which means it can be used to treat haemorrhoids and varicose veins and as a lymphatic and venous decongestant, whilst its cordial effect makes it useful for cardiac fatigue. Price (2007) cites it as being a possible therapeutic for lumbago, neuralgia, and sciatica. On an emotional level, Sandalwood has traditionally been used to help people through the transition between life and death. It may therefore be used in the treatment of terminally ill people and to help those who care for them. It may also help at other times of transition.

**Cautions:** Internal ingestion can lead to kidney damage. Also, this tree is under pressure and therefore should only be used when ethically sourced.

## Sandalwood, Western Australian (Santalum spicatum)

**Family:** Santalaceae

Sandalwood grows throughout most of W. Australia. A small ever-green tree, with sparse leaves at crown and irregular branching of crown. The bark is rough, fibrous, and furrowed on lower trunk and grey/blue and smooth on upper trunk and branches. The sapwood is pale, and the heart wood dark brown. Historically used in traditional tropical medicine and perfumery for hundreds of years. Sandalwood was used in the UK, French, and Belgian pharmacopoeias from 1920–1940, until the advent of antibiotics. *Santalum spicatum* has analogous use to *Santalum album*. The oil is distilled from the heartwood and root ball.

**Constituents:** pre-$\alpha$-santalol compounds (9–10%), $\alpha$-santalol (21–28%), farnesol (4–7%), alpha bisabolol (4–5%), z-$\alpha$-bergamatol (5–6%), $\beta$-santalol (24–28%), bergamatol-like compounds (17–24%), lanceol-like compounds (2–3%).

**Actions:** Antimicrobial (against *Staphylococcus aureus, S. epidermis,* MRSA, *S. sapropyticus, S. pyogenes, S. dysgalaciae, S. pneumoniae, Arcanobacterium haemolyticum, Legionella preumophilia, Proprionibacterium acnes, Acinetobacter calcoaceticus, Candida albicans, Saccahromyces cerevisiae*). Sandalwood is better that Tea Tree against Staphylococcus and about the same against Candida, biocidal against *Trichomonas vaginalis*, anti-inflammatory (farnesol and $\alpha$-bisabolol). Inhibits replication of herpes simplex virus 1, antifungal, diuretic, expectorant, and a pulmonary and urinary antiseptic. No cautions or contraindications known. In Australia, Sandalwood is licensed for topical and inhalation use.

**Uses:** Acne, tinea, ringworm, athlete's foot, inflamed skin conditions, and skin care generally. Cystitis, bronchitis, dry cough, and sore throats. reputed to help calm mental chatter and meditation. Davis (1991) suggests it's use for spiritual and emotional healing, connecting the base and crown chakras, and activating the heart and throat chakras. Sandalwood is an aphrodisiac. Traditionally, the plant was used by Australian aborigines as a cough medicine, for colds and stiffness, sores, boils chest infections, rheumatism, constipation, and aches and pains.

## Spearmint (Mentha spicata/viridis)

**Family:** Lamiaceae

The oil is steam distilled from the flowering tops of the herb. It is a yellow to green colour, with a characteristic smell, familiar to all who chew gum. Grown mainly in USA, Hungary, Spain, Yugoslavia, Russia, and China.

**Constituents:** Monoterpenes; pinenes, limonene, phellandrene. Monoterpenols; linalol, menthol. Oxides; 1,8-cineole. Ketones (50–70%); l-carvone, pulegone, menthone.

**Actions:** Anti-inflammatory, antiseptic, antispasmodic, astringent, carminative, cephalic, cholagogue, digestive, diuretic, expectorant, febrifuge, hepatic, nervine, stimulant, stomachic, tonic.

**Uses:** Spearmint has similar uses to Peppermint, but is gentler in action, the principal ketone being carvone. It also has a stronger tropism towards the digestive system.

In can be used in skin care including acne, dermatitis, and congested skin. As an expectorant and mucolytic, it is used in the treatment of asthma, bronchitis, catarrh, sinusitis, colds, and flu. Spearmint is also used for fevers. Its action on headaches, migraine, and neurasthenia is not as strong as Peppermint, but it is a valuable nervine used for stress and fatigue. However, it comes into its own in the treatment of colic, dyspepsia flatulence, nausea, and vomiting. This is due in part to its action as a cholagogue.

**Cautions:** Although high in ketones, the principal ketone is carvone, which is considered non-toxic. Therefore, as long as it is used at proper dilutions and in a responsible way there are no contraindications.

## Spruce, Black (Picea mariana)

**Family:** Pinaceae

**Constituents:** Camphene, tricyclene, pinene, carene longifolene, longicyclene, cadinene, borneol, longiborneol.

**Actions:** Antifungal, anti-infectious, anti-inflammatory, antiparasitc, antispasmodic, endocrine balancer, immunostimulant, neurotonic.

**Uses:** Many of the uses are similar to those of Pine, so refer to that profile too. Spruce is effective against Candida infections and is also valuable as a fumigant or air antiseptic. It can help to reduce inflammation in the prostate. It is used to treat rheumatism and can support the adrenals, the thyroid, and immune function. It is a valuable neurotonic for asthenia and low energy. It helps to deepen the breathing and reduce mucus.

**Cautions:** Only use externally.

## *Ti Tree or Tea Tree (Melaleuca alternifolia)*

**Family:** Myrtaceae

The oil is not renowned for a particularly pleasant odour, but this can be moderated by blending, particularly with Lavender. Tea Tree is obtained by steam distillation of the leaves and twigs. The oil is clear to yellow and highly fluid. Take care to obtain the true oil, as there are 300 different plants known as Tea Tree in Australia, from different botanical families—such as *Leptospermum, Kuszea,* and *Baeker,* and the following *Melaleucas; leucadendron, viridiflora, viridiflora A, linarifolia, bracteata*. It used to be possible to obtain an oil with only 4% cineole, but not anymore. Since cineole and terpineol are from the same biosynthetic pathway, the more cineole the lower the monoterpenol level will be, making the oil less effective as a eubiotic.

**Constituents:** Monoterpenes; pinenes, terpinenes, para-cymene, limonene, terpinolene, thujene, sabinene, myrcene, phellandrenes, terpinolene. Sesquiterpenes; $\beta$-caryophyllene, aromadendrene, viridiflorene, cadinene, muurolene, bicyclogermecrene, gurjunene, calamenene. Monoterpenols; terpenenol-4, $\alpha$-terpineol, globulol, viridiflorol, cubenol. Oxides; 1,8-cineole (17%), 1,4-cineole.

**Actions:** Analgesic, antifungal, anti-infectious, anti-inflammatory, antiviral, anti-parasitic, antibacterial, mild expectorant, immunostimulant, neurotonic, phlebotonic, radio-protective.

**Uses:** It is useful against all fungal infections, including athlete's foot, candida, and ringworm. As a bactericide it can be used for abscesses, skin infections, intestinal infections, bronchitis, genital infections, sore throats, gum infections, sinusitis, and otitis, as well as acne and suppurating wounds. It was used in the First World War to treat wounds. It is particularly effective in that the constituents fight the infection and travel through the pus to the raw skin, where they speed up the healing process and, therefore, prevent the infection travelling. Tea Tree is effective in the treatment of cold sores and other herpes infections and for treating chicken pox and shingles (see Eucalyptus and Bergamot). It will help get rid of intestinal parasites. As an immunostimulant, Ti Tree been used in conjunction with Garlic to raise the T4 cell count of HIV positive individuals, but is also useful for anyone with lower immunity due to stress etc. As a neurotonic, it can help treat debility, depression, PMS, and anxiety. Its action on the circulatory system makes it helpful for varicose veins, haemorrhoids, and aneurysms, and here its analgesic effects are also useful. It can be used for the prevention of burns in radiotherapy, although Niaouli is reputed to be even better. It can also be used to prevent post-operative shock and add healing of surgical scars. After surgery massage can be used to continue application, or alternatively foot baths. In this case it is applied in high concentrations for about a fortnight before surgery. If used in baths and inhalations at the first signs of a cold or flu, it can often stop the infection in its tracks. Neat Tea Tree dabbed on spots and acne can be very effective, but is somewhat drying to the skin, so be sure to use a moisturiser as well.

Its action on debility and boosting the immune system may make it helpful in ME or after glandular fever. However, do bear in mind that full body massage may be too exhausting and eliminating for people in this situation, so other methods of use may have to be used. A more mundane use is in mouth care, a single drop can be applied to ulcers (although it tastes truly awful) and it can be applied to abscesses, until a dentist can be reached. I know of several people who have treated the infection with Tea Tree, without resorting to antibiotics. Tea Tree is stimulating and refreshing, so can be included in a shower gel or bath blend for morning use.

It is an energising oil that can be useful for treating exhaustion. Emotionally it is seen as cleansing and detoxifying, useful for clearing out unwanted thoughts and emotions and purifying.

**Cautions:** Occasionally Tea Tree may cause mild skin irritation if used undiluted. If this occurs discontinue use for a period of a month. It may then be used diluted in Lavender or a base oil. Also, use caution when adding it to the bath, as some individuals may find that high concentrations cause irritation. Having said that, I recently added 5 ml to the bath and found no detrimental effects, quite the contrary.

## Thyme (Thymus vulgaris)

**Family:** Labiatae/Lamiacae

There are about 400 different species of Thyme. The wild population Thyme can be varied in constituents. There are many chemotypes of Thyme, obtained from clonal populations, some of which occur naturally.

This is generally known as Thyme or Red Thyme oil (this is nothing to do with the colour of the flowers!). A rectified form is also widely available and is known as White Thyme. Whilst Red Thyme may occasionally be of use to aromatherapists, White Thyme should never be used in common with other adjusted oils.

The oil is steam or water distilled from the flowering tops and leaves. Sometimes the dried plant is used for distillation. An absolute is also produced for perfumery use. Mainly produced in Spain, also in France, Israel, Greece, Morocco, Algeria, Germany, and U.A.

**Constituents:** Monoterpenes; paracymene, terpinene, pinene, camphene, myrcene, limonene, terpinolene, thujene, carene, sabinene, phellandrene; Sesquiterpenes: $\beta$-caryophyllene. Phenols; thymol, carvacrol. Monoterpenols; borneol, linalol, terpineol-4, $\partial$-terpineol, geraniol. Sesquiterpenols; nerolidol. Ketones; camphor, thujone. Esters; linalyl acetate, terpinyl acetate, geranyl acetate. Oxides; 1,8 cineole, linalol oxides.

**Actions:** Anthelmentic, anti-oxidant, antiputrescent, antiseptic, antispasmodic, antibacterial, astringent, capillary stimulant, carminative, cicatrisant, dermocaustic, expectorant, digestive tonic, diuretic, hypertensive, mental stimulant and general tonic, nervine, parasiticide, rubefacient, stomachic, sudorific, vermifuge, warming.

**Uses:** The main action of Red Thyme is as an antiseptic—thymol is twenty times stronger than phenol but much less of an irritant. It can be used for acne, boils, and other skin problems. It also has a special affinity for the respiratory system, since this is its main route of excretion and therefore is used to treat bronchitis, sinusitis, coughs, colds, flu, catarrh, laryngitis, sore throats, tonsillitis, and asthma. It can also be used in mouthwashes for gum infections. As a digestive tonic it is indicated for sluggish digestion and some stomach infections (it was traditionally used in the form of the herb as a meat preservative). Also, for flatulence, dyspepsia, and diarrhoea—a tea would be more appropriate here. As a hypertensor it can be used for low blood pressure and poor circulation. It is a very stimulating oil which can be used for general debility and fatigue, as well as anxiety, depression, and possibly for insomnia (when a person is too exhausted to get to sleep). It is a diuretic, which can be used for the treatment of oedema and cellulite. It is also a valuable antiseptic for cystitis and urethritis.

As a warming oil, Thyme may be used to treat arthritis and rheumatism, as well as stiff joints. Also used for intestinal parasites, scabies, and lice.

**Cautions:** May irritate the mucus membranes and cause dermal irritation. Large quantities are toxic, therefore limit dose and length of treatment. Best avoided in pregnancy.

## Sweet or soft Thymes

**Constituents:** Monoterpenols linalol/geraniol 60–80% Esters geranyl/ linalyl acetate.

**Cautions:** Due to the high levels of geraniol the geraniol chemotype should be used with some caution. The linalol type aids delivery so perhaps should be avoided until the last two weeks of pregnancy.

**Actions:** Antiseptic, choleretic, anti-infectious, anti-inflammatory, anti-fungal, antispasmodic (linalol type), anti-viral, cardiotonic (geraniol), nervine, uterine, ophthalmic.

**Uses:** As an antiseptic, soft thymes can be used in the treatment of sore throats, bronchitis, sinusitis, otitis, tuberculosis and tonsillitis. The monoterpenols make them valuable for the treatment of acne, as they are also anti-inflammatory. They are also used for the treatment of cystitis, urethritis and vaginitis. As anti-fungal agents they are excellent for the treatment of thrush. Again, the anti-inflammatory Actions also make them useful for the treatment of dry or weeping eczema and psoriasis. They may also be used for the treatment of viral infections, including viral enteritis and verrucae or for people with a tendency to repeated viral infections. Other areas where they may be indicated are muscular rheumatism, bronchial spasm, fatigue and cardiac fatigue. Although they may be used for eye problems, only the floral waters should be used for such problems unless specialised knowledge. Their non-aggressive natural makes them more applicable to general use, and makes them appropriate for infants and frail people.

## Valerian (Valeriana officinalis var. angustifolium)

**Family:** Valerianaceae
Steam distilled essential oil is produced in France and the UK, also concrete and absolute. Related species *V. wallichi* from India and *V. officinalis var. latifolia* from Japan.

**Constituents:** Monoterpenes; *α*-pinene, and camphene. Sesquiterpenes; *β*-caryophyllene, azulene, fenchene. Alcohols; geraniol, α-terpineol, borneol, patchouli alcohol, valerianol. Esters; bornyl acetate, formiate, butyrate, bornyl isovalerate (thought to be responsible for odour and therapeutic effects), eugenyl isovalerate. Aldehydes; valerenal. Ketones; valeranone, ionone. Acids; isovaleric, acetoxyvaleric.

**Actions** (may be derived from internal use of herb): Anodyne, antidandruff, diuretic, antispasmodic, bactericidal, tranquilliser (depresses CNS, muscle relaxant, respiratory and motor activity), hypnotic, hypotensive, sedative, stomachic.

**Uses:** Muscle spasms, palpitations, heart pain, spasms, neuralgia, fevers, nervous indigestion, insomnia, nervousness, restlessness, tension, agitation, nervous headaches, panic attacks According to Penoel and Franchomme its main applications are for stress related conditions, tachycardia and fever, whilst the Indian variety is mainly useful for haemorrhoids and other varicosities as well as asthenia.

**Cautions:** Avoid in pregnancy, with children and babies, due to a possibility of sensitisation. Appears non-toxic and non-sensitising at normal dilutions. Overuse may cause lethargy.

## Vetivert (Vetiveria zizanoides)

**Family:** Poaceae

Steam distilled from the dried root of the grass. Cultivated in Reunion, the Philippines, the Comores, Japan, West Africa, and South America. The oil is mainly distilled in Java, Haiti, and Reunion. Traditionally the leaves are woven into matting and into the roof. This is said to protect the house from evil spirits. The plant is also used to protect animals from pests and is grown to prevent soil erosion. The aroma is somewhat heavy and smoky, but this becomes less noticeable when blended, especially with floral and citrus oils. The true oil is very thick—if it is mobile it has probably been rectified.

**Constituents:** Sesquiterpenes; etivene, vetiazulene, tricyclovetivene. Alcohols; vetiverol, bicyclovetiverol (12%), tricyclovetiverol (3%). Esters; vetiverol acetate. Ketones; vetiverones (7%). Acids; vetivenic acid, palmitic acid, benzoic acid.

**Actions:** Anti-infectious, circulatory tonic, emmenagogue, glandular tonic, immuno-stimulant, sedative.

**Uses:** As an anti-infectious oil, it is particularly useful for skin infections, such as acne, and also acts to boost the immune system in generalised infections. Although cited as an emmenagogue, it regulates the hormones, helping to overcome both oestrogen and progesterone imbalances. It has also been used for absent or scanty periods. Vetivert appears to have an action on both the pancreas and liver, helping to stimulate digestive secretions. It is also used for arthritis and urticaria. I have found it particularly useful for depression and insomnia, especially where people appear to have become 'ungrounded'. As a root oil it is profoundly grounding. Davis (1991) says that it balances all of the chakras and is very useful to protect the Solar plexus against oversensitivity. I have found this to be true for myself and others, applied before going into environments where there is likely to be a lot of negative feelings around. Although not mentioned by any other authors for this purpose, I have used it to clear the atmosphere in new environments.

**Cautions:** None known.

## Yarrow (Achillea millefolium)

**Family:** Asteraceae

Yarrow is steam distilled from the dried herb and grown in most temperate regions of the world—mainly distilled in Germany, Hungary, France, and Yugoslavia. Two oils are available; brown and blue, depending on the parameters of distillation. Its name comes from the fact that Achilles is said to have used it in battle for treating wounds and millefolium is due to the highly divided leaflets. The stalks are traditionally used for I Ching divination. There are several related species—Ligurie and Musk Yarrows are described below. *Achillea santolina* is used in Bedouin medicine and *Achillea ptarmica* or Sneezewort was a traditional medicine in Europe.

**Constituents:** Monoterpenes; pinenes (15%), camphene (up to 13%), sabinene, myrcene, terpinene, limonene, terpinene, terpinolene, cymene. Sesquiterpenes (highly variable depending on where it is grown); chamazulene (5–33%), dihydroazulenes, caryophyllene, germacrene. Monoterpenols; terpineol-4, borneol. Sesquiterpenols; cadinols. Oxides; 1,8-cineole (2–11%), caryophyllene oxide. Ketones; isoartemisia ketone (9%), borneone (2.9–16%), thujone. Esters; bornyl acetate (2.2%). Lactones; achilline. Phenols; eugenol.

**Actions:** Analgesic, anti-allergic, anti-catarrhal, anti-inflammatory, antipyrtetic, antiphologistic, antiseptic, antispasmodic, astringent, choleretic, cicatrisant, decongestant, diaphoretic, digestif, diuretic, emmenagogue, expectorant, febrifuge, hypotensor or possibly balances blood pressure, litholytic, vulnerary.

**Uses:** Yarrow herb is used for regulating fever, particularly when combined with Elderflower and Peppermint. It is also used to reduce heavy periods, one cup of strong infusion being taken each day. The oil is used to treat colds and catarrh, helping to reduce fever and expectorate phlegm. It can also be used for other febrile conditions. It has an affinity for the kidneys, being used for infections of the urinary system and also for stones. Yarrow can also be used to reduce inflammation of the prostate. Its anti-inflammatory and analgesic actions also make it valuable for the treatment of neuralgia, headaches, neuritis, sprains, arthritis, and rheumatism. As a choleretic, it can be used to treat liver deficiencies and poor or sluggish digestion, including constipation, colic, cramp, and flatulence. It also helps to relieve diarrhoea and aids detoxification, as well as treating haemorrhoids. As a vasodilator it can be used to treat hypertension. As well as being used for heavy periods it can be used for absent periods and for period pain. As a vulnerary it can be used to treat varicose ulcers and wounds. It can treat skin conditions such as acne, burns, warts, eczema and other skin irritations, inflammations, scars, and acts as an astringent for the skin and scalp. It also promotes hair growth and perspiration in the form of herbal poultices.

**Cautions:** Due to ketones, do not use on pregnant women, or children under twelve. May be neurotoxic and abortifacient. Can cause sensitivity. Some confusion as to whether or not it contains ketones, due to the fact that there are over fourteen species of *Achillea*, which are virtually inseparable.

## Ylang Ylang (Cananga odorata var. genuina)

**Family:** Annonaceae

Ylang Ylang oil can vary widely in its composition. It is extracted from the flowers of a tall tropical tree—the name means flower of flowers. Although the trees bear flowers of pink, mauve or yellow, the yellow flowers are regarded as the best. Immature green flowers do not yield a good quality oil, neither do flowers that are bruised during harvesting. Since the flowers are handpicked and such care must be taken during harvesting, it is only reasonable to expect the oil to be more expensive than some of those that are easier to produce, such as Lemon or

Rosemary. The freshly picked flowers are steam or water distilled. The distillation may be a long process and several grades of oil are available. The best is the 'complete', which contains the entire distillate. The next grade is 'extra', I, then II and III. The complete, extra, and third grades are the most widely used. An inferior oil is produced from a close relative and is commonly known as Cananga oil. An absolute and a concrete are also produced by solvent extraction for the perfumery industry. The oil is a pale to deep yellow, with a slightly oily or viscous consistency. The odour is sweet and spicy, with a floral side to it—some find it rather sickly. Native to Indonesia and the Philippines and mainly produced in Madagascar, Reunion, and the Comores.

**Constituents:** Monoterpenes; pinenes. Sesquiterpenes; farnesene, $\gamma$-cadinene (6–17), $\beta$-caryophyllene (15–22%), germacrene (15–25%), humulene (1–2%). Monoterpenols; linalol (11–30%), geraniol, nerol, benzyl alcohol. Sesquiterpenols; farnesol. Phenols; eugenol. Esters (15%); geranyl acetate, benzyl acetate, benzyl benzoate, methyl benzoate, methyl salicylate (1–10%), methyl anthranilate, cresyl acetate, farnesyl acetate benzyl salicylate. Phenyl methyl ethers; para cresyl methyl ether, safrole, methyl eugenol.

**Actions:** Anti-diabetic, antiseptic, antispasmodic, aphrodisiac, anti-seborrhoeic, calming, euphoric, hypotensor, tonic, reproductive tonic, sedative.

**Uses:** The primary uses of Ylang Ylang are as a skin care oil and for anxiety and stress-related problems, especially hypertension. For skin care it has traditionally been used in the Philippines to make a hair pomade, including coconut oil. This was used to improve the health of the hair and scalp and encourage glossy, luxuriant growth. It can also balance sebum production and soothe irritated skin. Apparently, it soothes insect bites as well, although I would not think of this as a first choice. For anxiety and panic attacks the oil is excellent. It slows the breathing and lowers the heart rate and blood pressure, helping to induce physical relaxation. It can help with full blown panic attacks, but also with day-to-day stress symptoms, such as insomnia, depression, lowered libido, and nervous tension. It may also help with hypertension as an arterial hypotensive, palpitations, and tachycardia. Two other areas in which it appears to help is in the control of diabetes and in lessening the frequency and severity of epileptic seizures, although such cases can only be undertaken with the full consent of the patient and the physician thereof. Personally, I have seen several people benefit from the use of this oil with epilepsy, especially where stress is a major trigger.

**Cautions:** High percentages have been shown to cause skin irritation and allergic reactions in sensitive individuals. It may also cause extreme stupor in individuals with low blood pressure. Over exposure occasionally causes headaches and nausea.

*CHAPTER 9*

# It's all about the base-carrier oils, macerated oils, and creams

This chapter covers some brief notes on the properties and uses of bases; carrier oils, macerated oils, creams, and hydrosols. The selection of bases is a highly individual choice. I often use organic olive oil due to the fact it is a reasonable price, easily accessible and well tolerated by most people. However, there is a large range of beautiful oils available so one's choice depends on how much one wishes to spend, what oils your preferred supplier(s) stock, the shelf life of the oil and one's views on sustainability (is it locally produced). Do bear in mind that most cold-pressed oils have a short shelf life, especially once opened. It is, therefore, better to choose a small range to start off with and then expand this depending on how much one is using and what is most suitable for your patient/client range.

Vegetable oils may be used internally and externally for their therapeutic properties. To derive the best benefit, it is best to use cold pressed and unrefined oils. Oils that are prepared in this way contain the highest levels of vitamins, minerals, essential fatty acids, and lecithins. They have not been subjected to high temperatures and chemical processes to remove their natural pigments and aromas, as is the case with refined oils.

When an oil is refined, the heating encourages oxidation and the formation of free radicals and hydroperoxides. These molecules can cause extensive damage to the tissues and cells of the body and are thought to accelerate the aging process, as well as being implicated in oncogenesis. They should therefore be avoided in the diet and in the formulation of skin preparations.

Unrefined oils are normally high in essential fatty acids. These are required by the body to build healthy cell membranes, for healthy nerve and liver function, amongst other things. A lack of these in the diet can be a contributory factor to heart disease, cancer, and stress disorders, as well as weak nails, hair, and skin. The benefits of taking the right sorts of fatty acids into the body can include increased energy, greater resistance to heart disease, a reduction in inflammatory disorders, a stronger immune system, and improved condition of the hair, nails, and skin.

As well as protecting our complexions from aging, some vegetable oils can help reduce free radical damage and, therefore, reduce aging inside the body. Certain groups of fatty acids can also help control/balance cholesterol levels in the body and prostaglandin production. These will be explained below.

## Selecting oils for medicinal and dietary use

Always check that oils are labelled as cold pressed *and* unrefined. Cold pressed oils may have been subjected to further processing to remove the colour and odour. A good oil should be richly pigmented and have a distinct, but fresh odour.

Oils should not be prepared from roasted seeds or nuts. The exception is that some culinary oils are prepared from toasted seed, for example toasted sesame seed oil. Oils should be packaged in dark glass or metal to protect them from photo-oxidation and should carry a best before date. Their natural antioxidants mean that they should have a shelf life of at least nine months, but it is better to purchase small quantities to ensure that they are fresh.

The shelf life of oils is prolonged by storing in a cool, dark place. They may become slightly cloudy, but this is the sign of a good quality oil. Remember that the fixed oil from a particular species will not possess all the therapeutic properties of the whole herb. It is also a good idea to check that the oil is from the correct botanical species—for example, in the cosmetic industry much of the Carrot oil sold is in fact prepared from French Marigold, which gives a similar pigmentation, but different therapeutic properties.

Also remember that hydrogenated vegetable fats have been treated in such a way that they affect the body in the same way as saturated fats. It is therefore probably better to exclude them from the diet and from skin care.

## The nature of fats

Fatty substances can be divided into oils, fats, waxes, and lipids, which are collectively referred to as 'total lipids'. All these substances are insoluble in water, but will dissolve in each other e.g. beeswax and almond oil will form a solution when heated together.

We tend to think of oils as a viscous material that is thicker than water and acts as a lubricant. We think of waxes as being solid and harder and butters as being solid and soft. However, Jojoba 'oil' is in fact a wax, and cocoa butter is solid like a wax. Also, the consistency will depend on temperature, so that if jojoba is put in the fridge, it will become more solid and coconut oil (which we think of as a solid) will become liquid on a hot day.

Oils from biological sources are produced by the organism to perform specific functions. They provide heat insulation, protect organs, and are used as sources of energy and energy stores. Most of the fats that we use are energy stores laid down in the seed or nut to be used as a source of energy when the seed sprouts. Fats also provide building blocks for cells and are combined with protein to form the lipoprotein bilayer that encapsulates every cell.

## Fats sources

- Vegetable origins
- Animal origins
- Marine animal origin
- Micro-organisms
- Mineral sources—e.g. mineral oil and paraffin wax

In plant medicine we only use those of vegetable origin. From the nutritional point of view, we need to understand those of animal and marine origins too—even if you are vegetarian many of your clients will not be but may have enquiries about nutritional matters.

## Composition of fats

All fats are made up of triglycerides. These contain three fatty acids attached to a molecule of glycerol/glycerine, which is an alcohol. Glycerides are therefore esters, being made from an acid and an alcohol with any water removed.

As glycerol is trivalent (has three hands) it can hold onto three fatty acids. Therefore, triglycerides are the ones most often seen in natural oils. Mono- and di-glycerides do exist, but we do not need to concern ourselves with these at present.

In the same way that there are different types of acids in essential oils, there are different fatty acids. A triglyceride may have three of the same fatty acid or three different ones, or one of one type and two of another. The fatty acids may be saturated or unsaturated (see below) and, therefore, there are many different triglycerides that make up fats. This also means that it is difficult to analyse the glycerides present in a particular fat, so, oils are normally classified by their fatty acid composition.

**Saturated**—These contain no double bonds, which means that the carbon molecules have the maximum possible number of hydrogen molecules attached. They are usually solid at room temperature. They mainly occur in animal fats and solid vegetable fats such as coconut.

Examples of saturated fatty acids include; butyric (C4), caprylic (C8), lauric (C12), myristic acid (C14), palmitic acid (C16), and stearic acid (C18).

Palmitic acid is used to make creams and ointments. Stearic acid is used to make candles. High levels of saturated fatty acids in the diet may actually increase the level of low-density lipoproteins in the body (otherwise known as bad cholesterol!).

**Unsaturated**—contain a high proportion of fatty acid molecules with at least one double bond.

**Monounsaturated**—These contain one double bond, which is sufficient to make them liquid at room temperature. However, they often go cloudy if the temperature drops, since they have a higher melting point than polyunsaturated fats. They are found in animal, fish, and vegetable oils, particularly olive and palm oil.

For example, oleic acid (C18 with a double bond between the 9th and 10th carbon atoms). Written as 18: 1,9 C.

**Polyunsaturated**—These contain several double bonds and are therefore the most liquid. They are found in vegetable oils, including sunflower, safflower, and corn oil. As well as being important energy sources, it has already been mentioned that fatty acids are used structurally in the body. They also give rise to hormone-like substances, known as prostanoids and leukotrienes. Some of the fatty acids needed for these functions cannot be produced within the human body and are therefore an essential part of the diet. Linoleic and $\alpha$-linolenic acid are definitely in this class and arachidonic acid may also be.

## A brief word about cholesterol

Polyunsaturated fats have received much coverage as being useful in reducing 'harmful' low density lipoprotein cholesterol (LDLs), in the blood stream, which is the form that deposits plaques in the blood vessels and may lead to thromboses and heart attacks. However, there are two forms of cholesterol in the body: LDLs and HDLs (high density lipoproteins). Cholesterol is not bad in itself. Our bodies manufacture cholesterol in the liver and the less there is in our diet, the more we produce.

Cholesterol is used by the body to transport fats through our body fluids. It is also used as a raw material to manufacture hormones and is involved in keeping the fatty sheaths of our nerve cells in good condition. However, if our body cannot process its blood fats and cholesterol correctly, due to too many saturated fats, polyunsaturated fats and refined carbohydrates or insufficient monounsaturated fats and fibre, problems occur. It would appear that damage to blood vessels is more likely to be caused by refined carbohydrates and the LDLs are part of an inflammatory process and the body's attempt to heal the vessels. Cutting down on refined carbs and processed foods is what helps.

HDLs prevent cholesterol deposits in the arteries by transporting LDLs back to the liver from the body cells. There they can be converted into bile acid. In order for this process to occur, there must be a ratio of 1:5 of HDLs to LDLs. Polyunsaturated fats appear to reduce both LDLs and HDLs rather than maintaining the correct balance. Monounsaturated fats appear to maintain the correct balance, but only if they are taken in sufficient quantities. Therefore, the inclusion of olive oil, walnuts, and almonds in the diet is definitely desirable.

## Essential fatty acids and γ-linoleic acid

In theory, our bodies should be able to manufacture $\gamma$-linoleic acid from linoleic and linolenic acid. However, it is necessary to have sufficient linoleic acid in the diet to do this, and the modern diet often does not contain sufficient vegetables, oils, seeds, and pulses for this. Also, the metabolic process can be inhibited by too many saturated fats, or by insufficient zinc, magnesium, or vitamin B6. Other inhibitory factors include diabetes, viral infections, pregnancy, menopause, old age, excessive alcohol intake, and smoking. The recommended daily intake of essential fatty acids (EFAs) is 3% of our dietary calories or 5–6% in children and lactating women.

Gamma-linoleic acids are involved in the production of prostaglandins, hormone-like substances, which are produced throughout the body in response to certain stimuli, and are then rapidly broken down. They control the movement of matter between cells and control the transmission of nerve impulses.

Deficiency in EFAs leads to skin disorders, hair loss, and poor wound healing. Cell membranes also become less flexible, including those of the immune system, e.g. lymphocytes, so that EFAs may be necessary for a healthy immune system. They may also be useful for treating inflammatory diseases such as arthritis where cell rigidity may be a problem.

Prostaglandins are also derived from EFAs, particularly linolenic acid. They act as cell regulators. The amount produced in the body depends on enzymes converting the EFAs into prostaglandins, and therefore the amount produced is regulated if there are more than enough EFAs. However, if there are insufficient quantities the enzymes have no raw materials.

There are several types of prostaglandin, but prostaglandin 1 is especially important. It is involved in the functioning of the immune system and is also involved with other conditions, including hypertension and depression. When there is not enough of this prostaglandin there is more likely to be autoimmune disease, including multiple allergies. The body needs the natural unrefined form of linoleic acid to make it, which is called the *cis* form. If it is refined and hardened (changed into the *trans* form) as in margarine then the enzymes cannot use it and it will actually block their action. The same is also true of refined oils.

## The chemistry of fats

In the same way that essential oils are not oily, fatty acids are not fatty, they only become that way when combined into triglycerides. They are known as fatty acids because they were first isolated from fats. In common with essential oils, they are made up of carbon, hydrogen, and oxygen. As you will remember, carbon is able to form chains of varying lengths. You will also remember that substances that only contain carbon and hydrogen are called hydrocarbons and that the simplest one is methane. This is written as $CH_4$.

If two carbons form a chain then they will only be able to combine with six hydrogens, since each carbon atom forms four bonds, each carbon uses one of those bonds to join the neighbouring carbon, This substance is a gas and is called ethane. It is written as $C_2H_6$. Carbons can form straight chains as above, or branched chains, or they may form rings, as they do in many essential oil components. The different structures give different activities and are therefore classed into different groups of chemicals or similar molecules.

Fatty acids are classified as carboxylic molecules, or as being in the *carboxyl* group. This means that at the end of each chain there is a characteristic group—COOH. This should look familiar as it is also the characteristic group of the volatile acids found in essential oils and floral waters.

It is the carboxylic group that gives acids their ability to dissolve in water. This is true of the acids found in essential oils, which is why they also occur in the floral water—they are hydrophilic [literally this means love (*philos*) water (*hydros*)]. On the other hand, hydrocarbons repel water, they are hydrophobic [afraid (*phobia*) of water].

When you have an acid with a short carbon chain, its behaviour is dictated by the carboxyl group and therefore it will readily dissolve in water. We are all familiar with acetic acid, which is the acid in vinegar and know that this easily mixes with water. This is because it only contains two carbons.

However, in acids where there is a longer chain of carbons (eight or more), the carbon chain starts to have an effect on the behaviour of the molecule and you end up with a molecule which has one end that loves water and another which hates it. If it is added to water, it will form a layer with the carboxyl end sticking into the water and the hydrophobic end sticking out, trying to keep it's toes dry. This is called *surface activity* and this property is used in making soaps, detergents, and emulsions (that is creams and lotions). It is also involved in the way that our cell membranes are formed, but if you want to know about that look at a physiology book. · Palmitic and stearic acids are the main fatty acids used in making soaps.

You will notice that most fatty acids have an even number of carbons. Most commonly they contain 16–18, but there are some with 12–24. Shorter chain fatty acids are found in milk (6–8).

## Refining and processing

It would be wonderful if we could simply press our own oils from fresh olives, sunflower seeds, linseeds, rosehip seeds, and so forth, but this tends not to be practical for most of us. If we were making our own carrier oils then, hopefully, we would use the best produce, without blemish, press it while fresh and use it immediately. However, we are limited to buying what is available. It has already been mentioned that refined oils are not ideal, but why are they produced?

Oils are used for many things, including the manufacture of food, soap, paint, varnish, lubricants, and plastics. Production of such products is generally carried out by vast multinational organisations. Sometimes these companies own the production plantations, the shippers, millers, and even the byproduct industries. Oil business is big business.

When oils are produced on a large scale it often means that the poor quality seeds and nuts are used, since the better quality produce are sold for eating—e.g. almonds. The crop may be stored for a long time and shipped large distances before being milled, so that it will already have started to deteriorate. The finished product is expected to have a long shelf life, exposed to light and warmth on the shop shelf. It is expected to be identical from batch to batch and when opened may be used slowly. This is why oils are refined and you can see that it has something in common with the essential oils that are processed for the perfumery market, where the therapeutic applications are not under consideration. Refined oil is 'pure', bland, stable, and uniform. When the oils are processed, they are split into fractions and become very profitable for the producer.

During refining the following steps occur, from the nut/seed to the end product:

- The seed is cleaned and isolated from other matter.
- The seeds are ground to rupture the cell walls.
- Steam pressure is applied to further break the microscopic cells open. The seed is in effect cooked.
- An expelbo (large pressing plate), which may be heated or unheated (cold pressed), forces the oil out of the starting material and through a filter. This is the finest virgin oil. Other claims such as extra virgin have little meaning.

- The residual cake still contains oil. Therefore, the cake is broken into flakes.
- The flakes are put into a solvent extractor. They are washed with petrol and an oil/solvent solution results. It is then distilled and the petrol evaporated off. The left over meal usually is used as animal fodder (not exactly great food for the animals).

At this stage the oil can then be refined. There are three stages to the process. Natural acids are removed, the colour is 'adjusted' and the smell/taste has to be 'improved'.

- Caustic acid is used to remove fatty acids, including the essential ones. This is the basis of soap making.
- Fuller's earth or carbon power is used to remove the colour.
- High pressure steam is used to remove any odour.

When making margarine an additional step of hardening or hydrogenation is carried out. The oil is heated with a catalyst, such as nickel and hydrogen gas is bubbled through it. This alters the unsaturated fats into the *trans* form. The human body breaks down fatty acids using enzymes. These cleave off two carbon atoms at a time to give acetyl co-enzyme A. When the carbon chain's shape is altered from the natural *cis* form to the *trans* form then enzymes are unable to do this and, therefore, they are not broken down totally. The partially metabolised remains are treated as toxins or waste to be eliminated, which makes you wonder whether margarine really is better for you than butter.

## For and against refining

As holistic practitioners, we should always use products as near to nature as possible, providing they are in good condition. Processed oils and fats are far from close to nature. However, from the moment of harvesting and milling the surface area is exposed to oxygen and the fats will start to oxidise, producing free radicals. Natural oils deteriorate faster. Acidity levels may also be altered, dropping below 5.5—the pH of our skin. Therefore, unrefined oils should be bought in amounts that will not be left sitting around. Any oil that smells rancid or 'off' should be thrown away. Unfortunately, people do not expect oils to smell, even when the aroma is delightfully nutty. I have heard therapists complain that unrefined sunflower oil 'smells nutty'. Some oils with exotic names can have rather more unpleasant odours. I think the most amusing complaint I had was that unrefined avocado oil was dark green (the refined oil is colourless) and smelt of bacon rashers. Either this person had been a vegetarian for many years, but had never eaten an avocado, or their local butcher was selling a very strange sort of bacon.

Within the oil trade, the quality of the raw material is reflected by the prices it commands and the industry that uses it. For example, Camellia oil comes in four grades: pharmaceutical, cosmetic, cooking, and then industrial. Each grade has its price structure and obviously the first two grades will be the most expensive. As with essential oils, it is possible to get low priced versions of even the most exotic base oils, but they were originally intended for making things like paint and varnish!!

The more exotic oils are not usually available in the lower grades outside their country of origin as exporting them is not worth the return. Outside of Japan, Camellia oil is little used in cooking. Its main application is as an excipient for direct injections of minerals and vitamins.

## Choosing base oils

The simplest choice is between a thin oil and a thick oil—i.e. those that sink in quickly and those that do not. However, one should also consider whether the oil is being used solely as a carrier or as part of the treatment? Whenever skin damage, inflammations, immune deficiencies, or plain neglect of the skin due to stress are involved, it is always advisable to make informed choices and use the most appropriate vegetable oil to form part of the treatment.

The following oils are mainly produced for industrial uses and therefore should be selected carefully to ensure that the correct grade is being obtained.

- Soya bean
- Peanut
- Cottonseed
- Sunflower
- Olive
- Sesame
- Coconut

- Palm
- Palm kernel

Also, if a person has an allergy to the plant that the oil is obtained from then it is not the right oil to use for them.

## Almond (Prunus amygdalus var. dulcis)

**Family:** Rosaceae
**Dilution:** 100%
**Composition:** 24–26% linoleic, 65–68% oleic, 6–8% palmitic, 2% stearic.
Sweet Almond should be used as Bitter Almond may contain traces of cyanide. In fact, the fixed oil is normally produced from Sweet Almond, whereas an essential oil, smelling of marzipan, is produced from the Bitter Almond. Almond oil is a pale yellow colour when cold pressed but relatively odourless. It contains vitamins E, D, A, B1, 2, and 6. It is used for its emollient properties in cosmetics and pharmaceutical ointments. It is also useful for strengthening the nails, by massaging around the cuticle and nail bed and as a hair conditioner. It may be used as a cleanser and has a certain ability to screen out U.V.

Ground almonds can be used as a gentle exfoliant and skin cleanser. Used internally, Almond oil actually contains more monounsaturated fat than olive oil and is therefore even more effective against cholesterol build up. The oil, ground almonds and whole nut can be included in the diet. It also has laxative properties, so be aware of this 'side effect' if taking it internally.

## Apricot kernel (Prunus armeniaca/Armeniaca vulgaris)

**Family:** Rosaceae
**Dilution:** 100%
**Composition:** 3–7% palitic, 0.5–1.5% stearic, 65% oleic, 28% linoleic.
Apricot kernel oil contains high levels of polyunsaturated fats and moderate levels of essential fatty acids. Its vitamin content is minimal. This oil is pale yellow in colour and is not as stable as almond. However, it has a light silky texture and absorbs easily into the skin. It can be very helpful for premature aging, sensitive, inflamed, and dry skins. Peach kernel is very close in its properties and the two can be interchanged. They are both similar to Almond oil. In the past they were cheaper,

but this is no longer the case. Therefore, Almond oil is probably the best choice when looking for these qualities.

## Avocado (Persea americana)

**Family:** Lauraceae
   **Dilution:** 10–25%
   **Composition:** 10–20% linoleic, 2% linolenic, 1% myristic, 60–90% oleic, 4–12% palmitic, 3% palmitoleic, 2% stearic. Vitamins A, B1, B2, D, and E, panthothenic acid, potassium, and lecithin.

Unrefined avocado oil is a deep green due to large quantities of chlorophyll and has a distinctive nutty aroma. Avocado penetrates deep into the skin, making it excellent for severely undernourished or stressed skin. It is also very soothing and softening and can be used for eczema. It has a natural ability to block UV light. However, be aware that with the erosion of the ozone layer vegetable oils will probably not give sufficient sun screening, especially in regions with high ambient light levels. If it is cheap then it is likely to be a maceration of the pulp in sunflower oil. Avocado pulp produces a very thick, fatty oil (4–40%), depending on the season. The pure oil is produced by expressing the dried pulp. It has highly variable amounts of sterols, hydrocarbons, volatile acids, amino acids, and very high levels of vitamin D. One constituent, biscatechin, condensed flavonol, has been reported to have antitumour activity. The pure oil is useful for arthritis and sclerosis of the skin.

## Blackcurrant (Ribes nigrum)

**Family:** Grossulariaceae
   **Dilution:** 10–25%
   **Composition:** 45–60% linoleic, 15–20% linolenic, 1% oleic, 2% stearic, 20% G.L.A. Traces of vitamins and minerals.
   For properties see Rose hip oil.

## Borage/Star flower (Borago officinalis)

**Family:** Boraginaceae
   **Dilution:** 10%
   **Composition:** 31–42% linoleic, 19–25% linolenic, 10–20% G.L.A.
   See Rose hip for properties.

## Coconut (Coco nucifera)

**Family:** Palmae
   **Dilution:** 100%
   **Composition:** 44% lauric, 2% linoleic, 17% myristic, 7% oleic, 11% palmitic, 6% stearic.
   This oil is a white solid or a translucent liquid, depending on the amount of processing. The fat from the flesh is heat extracted and then may be deodorised. Only the unfractionated oil should be used. It has a certain sun screening ability. It is also valuable for making body oils and creams, since it is solid at room temperature.

## Corn/maize (Zea mays)

**Family:** Graminaeae
   **Dilution:** 100%
   **Composition:**
   This oil contains high levels of polyunsaturated fats and omega 6 essential fatty acids in its natural state. However, it is mainly produced by heat extraction. The fresh oil contains large amounts of vitamin E, however, it degenerates quickly and the oil has a short shelf life.

## Evening primrose seed (Oenothera biennis)

**Family:** Onagraceae
   **Dilution:** 10–25%
   **Composition:** 70–79% linoleic, 10% linolenic, 1% myristic, approximately 9% GLA.
   The GLAs in Evening Primrose oil are of a different isomer to those in Blackcurrant seed and Rose hip oil, but the same as those in Borage. It would appear that those in Rose hip are more bioactive. This oil is reputedly helpful for eczema and psoriasis. It is useful for all types of scar tissue. Used on dry skin, it will improve the skin's water retaining properties. This is due to the essential fatty acids helping to regenerate healthy cell membranes. Internally it is also helpful for PMS symptoms, including cramps, water retention, swollen and tender breasts. It may also be helpful for menopausal problems, inflammatory conditions, such as osteo and rheumatoid arthritis, and irritable bowel

syndrome. It has also been used to treat alcohol-induced liver damage, schizophrenia, anorexia nervosa, Parkinson's disease, hyperactivity, cystic fibrosis and multiple sclerosis, where it restores red blood cell mobility and possibly helps delay deterioration of the myelin sheaths. It lowers blood cholesterol. Note that the only effect from external application is benefit for dry and irritated skin. I have found Evening Primrose oil to be particularly useful for reducing the redness and itching of psoriasis, eczema, dermatitis, and other skin conditions. It can also be used for itchy skin due to hormonal changes in pregnancy and menopause.

### Grapeseed (Vitis vinifera)

**Family:** Vitaceae
  **Dilution:** 100%
  **Composition:** 5–11% palmitic, 3–6% stearic, 12–20% oleic, 69% linoleic.
  The unrefined oil is extremely high in polyunsaturates. However, it is not generally available since it has a bitter taste and therefore does not appeal to the average palate. Even the refined oil has a pale green colour. Although it is readily absorbed into the skin, perhaps its refined nature makes it less ideal than some other choices. Although only anecdotal, I have had several reports of practitioners developing a form of dermatitis with prolonged exposure. A suitable cheap alternative is unrefined sunflower oil, which is a joy to work with.

### Hazel nut (Corylus avellana)

**Family:** Corylaceae
  **Dilution:** 25–100%
  **Composition:** 16% linoleic, 54% oleic, 2% palmitic, 3% stearic. The unrefined oil is a golden yellow with a fresh nutty aroma. If the oil is dark and smells toasted, it is probably from roasted nuts and is not suitable for use on the skin. Hazel nut oil is mildly astringent and therefore useful for oily or overactive skins. It also stimulates the circulation and is useful for inflammatory conditions. Its vitamin E content makes it fairly stable, and it is a light oil which penetrates the skin quickly. It is similar to Almond oil, but has quicker penetration.

## Jojoba (Simmondsia chinensis)

**Family:** Simmondsiaceae
   **Dilution:** 10–100%
   **Composition:** This is actually a liquid wax, rather than an oil, which makes it very stable. It is similar to Walnut oil in composition. The oil is obtained from the edible seeds of the plant and is 50% wax. It is odourless and clear, which makes it ideal for use with essential oils. It also is a valuable barrier to water. Environmentally, the plant can be used to reclaim desert and arid areas and, therefore, by using it we also help restore damaged areas of the planet. It shot to prominence as a vegetable substitute for sperm whale oil in the cosmetic industry. It is high in sterols, which gives it a non-greasy feel and gives a sheen to cosmetic formulae. Jojoba is rarely subjected to any refining processes. It has a similar composition to sebum in the skin and balances the amount produced, therefore useful for all skin types. It has a mild bactericidal action, which gives it a long shelf life and also means that it is therapeutically active in the treatment of acne. It also contains myristic acid which has anti-inflammatory properties.

## Linseed (Linum usitassium)

**Family:** Linaceae
   **Dilution:** 10–100%
   **Composition:** Linoleic, linolenic, omega-3 and 6, same as found in cod liver oil.
   This oil is valuable for boosting the immune system, treating inflammatory conditions, and moistening dry skin. It is also the fastest oil to penetrate the skin. Taking the oil internally can remove heavy metals, soothe itchy eyes, help with dryness of skin during menopause, treat constipation, and reduce the risk of thrombosis. The taste is rather bitter. It should be stored in the fridge.

## Macadamia nut (Macadamia integrifolia/ternifolia)

**Family:** Proteaceae
   **Dilution:** 25–100%
   **Composition:** 60% oleic, 18% palmitoleic, 6% linolenic/linoleic.

This is a light-coloured oil with little odour. It is a highly stable oil and is rapidly absorbed. It softens the skin and is non-irritant, making it useful for dry and mature skins. Palmitoleic acid is found in the skin of prepubescent children and its presence seems to delay the aging process. It also seems to reduce moisture loss.

## Neem (Azadirachta indica) Also known as margosa oil

**Family:** Meliaceae
  **Dilution:** 25–100%
  **Composition:** Azariachtin (triterpenoid), Nimbin (tripepenoid), Palmatic 13%, Stearic 24%, Oleic 62%, Linoleic 10%, Arachidic 3.2%, Myristic 2%.
  A viscous oil that requires warming for blending or pouring. It is traditionally used for skin and hair health, treating fungal skin infections and has a spermicidal action. It is considered to be good for treating skin infestations and adding lustre to the skin, hair and nails. It is also good for itchy skin.

## Olive (Olea europaea)

**Family:** Oleaceae
  **Dilution:** 10–100%
  **Composition:** 14–18% linoleic, 2% linolenic, 60–70% oleic, 10–18% palmitic, 2% stearic, Vitamin E.
  Good quality Olive oil is dark olive green and has a fruity rich aroma. It has an acidity level of less than 1%. Fine Olive oils are like fine wines, with specific regional oils. Its vitamin E content makes it useful for sore and inflamed skin, as well as sunburn. It is an emollient oil that is used pharmaceutically for severely dehydrated, chapped, or scaly skin conditions, including cradle cap. It is a valuable hair tonic, increasing the hair's tensile strength and adding shine. It is also used topically for rheumatic conditions and scarring or stretch marks. It also contains cyclarthanol, which blocks the absorption of high levels of cholesterol into the body. Its ratio of essential fatty acids is similar to human breast milk, making it suitable for small children. The vitamin E protects against free radical damage. As it contains anticoagulating agents, it reduces the risk of thrombosis. It cleanses the liver and stimulates the production

of bile, thereby acting as a digestive tonic and valuable aid to detoxifying programmes. It is also slightly antiseptic for balancing the gut flora. It also protects against gallstones, promotes pancreatic secretions, and may protect against stomach ulcers. Olive oil is one of the most stable oils at high temperatures.

## Palm kernel (Elaeis guineensis)

**Family:** Palmae
 **Dilution:** 25–100%
 **Composition:** 57% lauric, 2% linoleic, 13% oleic, 8% palmitic, 2% stearic. Coumarins and lactones.

This oil is yellowish green and solid at room temperature. The coumarin content has the effect of thinning the blood and the lactones are mucolytic. It is a warming oil and therefore should not be used in MS. However, it is valuable for viral and bacterial diseases as it stimulates macrophage activity. It can be used for haemorrhoids, diabetic ulcers, thread veins, enlargement of the prostate, weeping acne, and eczema. However, much Palm kernel oil does not come from sustainable and environmentally sound sources.

## Passionflower (Passiflora incarnata)

**Family:** Passifloraceae
 **Dilution:** 10–25%
 **Composition:** Linoleic acid.

This oil has a deep yellow colour and no distinct aroma. The oil is usually warm pressed but unrefined. It is useful on dry and stressed skin conditions, including eczema and psoriasis. Note that the oil does not have the same properties as the herbal preparation and, therefore, does not have any action on insomnia.

## Peanut (Arachis hypogaea)

**Family:** Leguminosae
 Peanut oil is usually highly refined so avoid. Also best avoided due to the prevelance of peanut allergies.

## Rosehip (Rosa rubiginosa)

**Family:** Rosaceae
  **Dilution:** 10–25% dilution.
  **Composition:** 33% linolenic, 45% linoleic, 15% oleic, 2% stearic, 4% palmitic, vitamins A and E.

This oil is a deep golden orange/yellow. It's GLA content means that it helps restore cell membranes. It is also useful for cauterised skin, burns, and sunburn. Its regenerative properties make it useful for dry or devitalised skin, dry acne, eczema, helping scars, stretch marks, and thread veins. It is reputed to reduce hyperpigmentation. Other actions of GLAs make it useful for auto immune diseases-including multiple sclerosis, liver congestion, insufficient digestive secretions, hypertension, thromboses, and hyperactivity in children, all of these are only with internal use. Also see Blackcurrant, Borage, and Evening Primrose oil.

## Safflower (Carthamus tinctorius)

**Family:** Compositae/Asteraceae
  **Dilution:** 100%
  **Composition:** 60–90% linoleic, 0.5% linolenic, 10–14% oleic, 6% palmitic, 3% stearic. Also, Omega-6 fatty acids.

In its unrefined state, Safflower oil is a rich yellow/orange with little odour. It is an easily absorbed oil which is nourishing for the skin and fairly inexpensive! May be especially useful for sensitive, dry, or stressed skin.

## Sesame (Sesamum indicum)

**Family:** Pedaliaceae
  **Dilution:** 100%
  **Composition:** Linoleic, monounsaturates.

This oil has a light odour and amber colour. Do not use the variety produced from roasted seeds except in stir frys. It's light texture and astringent properties make it ideal for massage and it reputedly does not stain the towels. It acts as a sunscreen, filtering out about 30% UV It may also be helpful for rheumatism, arthritis, psoriasis, and eczema.

Its composition gives it a long shelf life. Internally it is reputed to strengthen the lungs and act as an anti-inflammatory.

## Soybean (Glycine max)

**Family:** Leguminosae
Soy bean oil is normally refined. May also increase skin sensitisation on some individuals. Mainly produced for the industrial market so should be avoided.

## Sunflower (Helianthus anuus)

**Family:** Compositae/Asteraceae
**Dilution:** 100%
**Composition:** 50–70% linoleic, 20–40% oleic, 3–10% palmitic, 2–10% stearic. This oil has a deep yellow colour with a mild nutty aroma. It is useful for skin diseases, bruising, and leg ulcers. It is easily absorbed and is an inexpensive general-purpose oil. Used in the diet, it is easily digested and is traditionally thought be good for asthmatics.

## Tamanu (Caulophyllum inophyllum)

**Family:** Guttiferae
**Dilution:** 2–10% dilution.
**Composition:** Terpenic essences, benzoic and oxybenzoic acid, vitamin F, lipids, glycerides and saturated fatty acids, calophyllolide, calophyllic acid, coumarin derivatives, phosphoro-amino acids.

This oil is prepared from the seeds and berries of the plant. The berries and the cold pressed or infused oil are used in traditional medicine in Madagascar and Tahiti. The Madagascan preparation is referred to as 'foraha' and is mainly used in hair care preparations. In Tahiti the oil is used for a wide range of conditions; it is said to increase the oxygen circulation to the capillaries, rejuvenating tissues and aiding detoxification. It is used to treat an array of skin ailments including ulcers, atonic wounds, shingles, scars, eczema, burns, and surgical wounds. However, it should be used at low concentrations, since it can irritate sensitive or damaged skin. It has also been used to treat haemorrhoids, sciatica, and rheumatism. Tamanu has also been used to treat neuritis caused by leprosy. It has an antibiotic action, but is very warming on the skin. It should not be used on people with multiple sclerosis.

## Wheatgerm (Triticum vulgare)

**Family:** Graminae
  **Dilution:** 10–25% dilution
  **Composition:** 10% linolenic, 28% oleic, 14% palmitic, 3% stearic. This oil is high in vitamin E (about 190 mg in 100 g), provitamins A and D, lecithin.

The oil is a deep rich orange and has a strong odour. It has antioxidant properties that protect the double membrane of cells and help in scarring, stretch marks, and aging. It is also considered to improve the elasticity of blood vessels. Due to its rich odour and sticky texture, it is normally used diluted in another oil. In cases of people with wheat sensitivity, it may be better to substitute a vitamin E oil.

## Vitamin E

Vitamin E oil is a preparation of isolated vitamin E (normally $\alpha$-tecopherol) in sunflower oil. The highest concentration available is 4% at present.

## Solid fats

**Cocoa butter** is emollient, highly stable, and does not easily become rancid. It is quickly absorbed. It is solid at room temperature and therefore useful for creams. It melts at body temperature and is therefore used to make pessaries and suppositories.

  **Carnauba wax** has a high melting point, is non-toxic, and dermatophilic. Used in lip balms and a useful alternative to beeswax for vegans.

  **Beeswax** contains essential oils which give it its honey aroma. It does not get digested when eaten. It is dermatophilic and healing to the skin and is traditionally chewed like chewing gum to relieve sinus congestion.

## Macerated oils and herbal creams

Macerated oils are an infusion of a therapeutically valuable plant in a bland oil such as olive, sunflower, or almond. Traditionally, the plant material is placed in a clear glass container, covered in oil and left in the sunlight (or a hot press) for 2–3 weeks. If the oil is not sufficiently saturated at this point, it may be filtered off and poured over a fresh batch of plant material. During this process active constituents diffuse into the carrier. They can be prepared at home, and there is an alternative hot method, where the herb is placed into a double boiler and covered with oil, then heated gently for 2–3 hours, and this is a better method for some species such as Chickweed *Stellaria media* which only produce a therapeutically active oil from fresh plant material. Herbal creams are traditionally made from the macerated oil, but may also contain the tincture or infusion of the herb.

## Uses and applications

They are usually used externally and may be incorporated into a blend or used to make ointments and lotions. Again, note that some of the properties are only from internal usage. It is particularly important to note that an infused oil does not necessarily possess all the characteristics of the whole herb, or the essential oil. As with all botanical preparations, always check the botanical name since substitutions and adulterations occur. Note that infused oils may contain Wheatgerm oil as a preservative and this may make them unsuitable for people with wheat allergy.

As they are prepared by using sunlight, they would be stored in a cool, dark place in order to get the best shelf life. Although many infused oils contain Wheatgerm as a preservative, they are probably best used within a year so buy small quantities, and make sure they are supplied in dark glass bottles. Alternatively make your own.

## Properties and uses of specific oils

**Arnica** (*Arnica montana*) is prepared from the flowers. Its main action is as an antiphlogistic and capillary tonic in bruising, sprains, rheumatic pain, and phlebitis. This herb is highly toxic when taken internally and the oil/cream should not be applied to broken skin. Daisy infused oil is not widely available commercially but has all the same actions without the toxicity issues. We find Daisy superior in action and therefore recommend making this one, especially as it is more local.

**Calendula** (*Calendula officinalis*) is produced from the fresh or dried flowering heads. This oil contains sterols, flavonoids, and the essential oil (which is difficult, if not impossible, to obtain by distillation).

Being astringent and anti-inflammatory, this oil is particularly useful for its healing properties on scarred and damaged skin. It is also used in the treatment of inflamed skin conditions. It is therefore used for nappy rash, chapped or cracked skin, dry eczema, varicose veins and leg ulcers, haemorrhoids bed sores, bruises, chilblains, cracked nipples, thread veins, bruises, neuralgia, fungal infections of the skin, cuts, and grazes. The tincture is also used externally for the treatment of varicose veins and cold sores. It is not to be confused with macerated oils from other marigolds from *Tagetes minuta* or *glandulifera*.

**Carrot** (*Daucus carota*) oil is prepared from the root of the carrot, and is rich in $\beta$-carotene, as well as vitamins B, C, D, and E. It is used for burns and inflamed conditions. It is also reputed to lessen free radical damage and therefore slow the aging process. Make sure it is the true oil and not from *Tagetes sp*. It is very orange and will stain towels and clothes.

**Chamomile** (*Anthemis nobilis* or *Matricaria recuctita*) oil is prepared from the flowers. It speeds healing and reduces swelling. It is used for treating teething, allergic skin reactions (unless allergic to the Asteraceae), anal and vulval irritation, and fungal infections.

**Chickweed** (*Stellaria media*) is prepared from the fresh herb, using the warm method. It is excellent for itchy and inflamed skin and is therefore used for eczema of all types, psoriasis and dermatitis. It is also used for drawing splinters, for insect stings, burns, and scalds.

**Comfrey** (*Symphytum officinale*) is prepared from the leaves and contains a protein called allantoin, which encourages healthy cell division. This makes it valuable for treating wounds, skin ulcers, fractures, sprains, strains of muscles, arthritic joints, inflamed bunions, soft tissue damage and joints. It also relieves itchy, rough skin, including psoriasis and eczema and aids the healing of burns. As an ointment or lotion, it can help relieve arthritic and rheumatic joints. Plantain leaf oil has similar properties.

**Daisy** (*Bellis perennis*) The best oils are prepared from the flowers but the whole plant can also be used. Ox Eye Daisy flowers can be used as a substitute. The oil can be prepared from fresh or dried flowers and is a lovely golden colour. It is vulnerary, astringent, anti-inflammatory, and cicatrisant. Daisy oil is of low toxicity so safe to use on broken skin. It is the best oil we have found for bruising (although Immortelle is a close second), sprains, and strains. It is also valuable for healing sunburn and sun damage to the skin and for a range of skin disorders. It is also safe to use on cuts and grazes—in this case we make a cream with the oil. Additionally, it is a tonic for blood vessels so can be used for varicosities, thread veins, and phlebitis. As an anti-inflammatory, it can help with rheumatism, arthritis, and gout.

**Hypericum/St. John's Wort** (*Hypericum perforatum*) is prepared from the whole flowering plant. One active constituent is hypericin, a deep red pigment. It also contains a volatile oil, glycosides, pectins, and rutin. It is particularly useful for nerve tissue damage and inflammation that occurs with sciatica, neuralgia, fibrositis, and Bell's palsy. It may also help with Parkinson's and MS. It is used for burns, ulcers, sores, bites, bruises, and to ease the discomfort of rheumatic and arthritic joints. It softens the skin and keeps it supple.

**Meadowsweet** (*Filipendula ulmaria*) is a familiar plant which grows in ditches throughout Ireland. The flowering tops are used to produce an oil which is traditionally used for arthritis and aches and pains (it was one of the first sources of aspirin). Perhaps best avoided by individuals sensitive to aspirin.

**Mullein** (*Verbascum thapsus*) is prepared from the tall flower spikes. This oil is antiseptic and astringent. It can therefore be used for haemorrhoids, wounds, and chilblains. It may also help relieve rheumatism and arthritis.

**Witch Hazel** (*Hamamelis virginiana*) is prepared from the bark. Being rich in tannins the cream is strongly astringent. It can therefore be used for haemorrhoids, bruises, and inflamed swellings. It also can relieve the pain of varicose veins.

# CHAPTER 10

# Hydrosols/hydrolats/aromatic waters

These are produced by steam distillation of plant material and contain the water-soluble constituents. Cohobation is sometimes used, meaning that the water passes through many batches of plant material, so that the distillate is highly concentrated and contains the active water-soluble components of the essence. Therefore, the hydrosol has some similar properties to the essential oil, but may also have properties of the parent species that are absent in the essential oil. In some species, there may be a commercially available hydrosol where no essential oil is available—e.g. Witch Hazel and Cornflower.

Hydrolats may also be prepared from non-aromatic plants, such as oak, beech, and fern. The main groups of molecules which dissolve are the hydroxylic alcohols and acids, which give hydrosols their anti-inflammatory and mildly antiseptic actions. It is these suspended or dissolved particles that give the hydrolat its therapeutic action, and the first twenty litres are the best for therapeutic purposes.

Hydrolats should not contain preservatives, therefore they have a short shelf life, unless cared for properly. They may last up to two years, if stored in a cool, dark place. If they contain small particles or 'bloom' it does not mean they have gone off, but need to be filtered. Home brew filters are ideal. You will be able to smell if they are 'off', but remember that they are 'living' substances, so their aroma may alter slightly after purchase.

## Uses and applications

- Cosmetically as cleansers and toners
- As an alternative to water in the formulation of moisturisers, creams, and lotions
- Facial steaming and inhalations, either neat or diluted
- Foot baths, sitz baths, and full body baths (one litre is recommended by some authorities for a full bath!)
- In the preparation of compresses and poultices
- Sponging (especially in fevers, or for those requiring 'blanket baths' or spraying the skin and hair)
- When the skin is too damaged to touch, working on the elderly and very frail e.g. in hospices and for infants
- Washing out orifices—e.g. the vagina
- In humidifying devices instead of ordinary water, or you could devise your own
- In hot weather or centrally heated environments, I keep a spray bottle of hydrolat with me to spray over the face, neck etc. to keep me cool (in every sense of the word!)
- They may be taken internally and used in cooking. For internal usage about one teaspoon is added to a cup of water

The following are the main cited applications, but try experimenting with them:

Bay Laurel **Laurus nobilis** may be used in warm compresses for nerve pain and used for its antiseptic properties in bacterial skin infections.

Clary Sage **Salvia sclarea** is useful for congested, irritated or sensitive skin. It is especially useful for mature skin. It may be used as a toner, facial steam, or mist.

Cornflower **Centaura cyanus** main uses are for irritated eyes or skin. It has a cooling action.

**Eucalyptus globulus**—as with the essential oil, it is particularly useful as an inhalation or warm compress for respiratory infections.

Elderflower **Sambucus nigra flos** is used in eye and skin lotions. It is mildly astringent and stimulating, and therefore used in compresses for bruises, sprains, and chilblains. It is useful for whitening and softening the skin and preventing blemishes and is also popular as an aftershave to astringe and close the pores. It is used in baths, inhalations, and foot-baths for colds and influenza.

Immortelle *Helichrysum italicum* is excellent for treating bruising, open wounds, abscesses, and broken capillaries. It is also used for colds, sinus inflammation and fevers and is sedative.

Jasmine *Jasminum officinale* is used in inhalations for coughs and sore throats and on eye pads for soothing itchy eyes, conjunctivitis. It is toning for mature and greasy skin and is generally relaxing and calming.

Lavender *Lavandula angustifolia* is good for all skin types and problems; especially eczema, sun/windburn, and babies' skin including nappy rash and as a wash for candida. It is used in inhalations for respiratory problems. It is balancing.

Linden, Lime flower *Tilia x europea* is useful as a nervine in foot or full baths. It is especially refreshing and relaxing sponged over the face and neck for headaches, including migraine.

Melissa *Melissa officinalis* is calming for irritated and allergic skin conditions and used in compresses for digestive spasms. It is sedative.

Myrtle *Myrtus communis* is soothing and healing for the skin, used in inhalations for respiratory problems and to calm the nerves.

Neroli *Citrus aurantium* **flos** is a digestive tonic, in compresses and internally, especially nervous indigestion. As cleanser and tonic, it is valuable for impure, sallow, sensitive, and scarred skin. It is very uplifting and helps to treat shock and trauma and relieve nervousness.

Peppermint *Mentha x piperita* is used in compresses for digestive disorders, including diarrhoea, cramps, indigestion, and colic. It is also used to treat seasickness, fevers, migraine, sinusitis, and sunburn. It is cooling and astringent, so useful for red complexions, broken veins, inflamed and infected skin. It is also analgesic and excellent as a foot spray to cool and deodorize tired feet. It can also be used as a spray to cool menopausal hot flushes.

Roman Chamomile *Anthemis nobilis* is soothing, antihistamine, and antiallergic. It is useful eyewash for hay fever, for dermatitis, eczema, nappy rash, healing wounds, and inflammation and in inhalations to relieve swollen sinuses and catarrh. It is sedative.

Rose *Rosa damascena* is used to treat Spider nevae (spider angiomas which are a type of telangiectasis), wrinkled skin, dermatitis, dehydrated, dry, broken, and sensitive skin. It is also used in eye baths and mouthwashes and is considered uplifting and sedative.

Rosemary **Rosmarinus officinalis** is a good astringent that stimulates the circulation. It is used as an aperitif and a tonic for the elderly. It is also a good antiseptic aftershave and for purifying congested skin.

Witch Hazel **Hamamelis virginiana** is used to treat haemorrhoids, bruises, and inflamed swellings, including varicose veins. Also used for open pores and congested skin.

There are many other hydrosols available and this is a fascinating area of therapeutics to explore.

# CHAPTER 11

# Oils for the body systems and specific conditions

## The respiratory system

**Asthma:** Benzoin, Cajeput, Clary Sage, Eucalyptus, Frankincense, Lavender, Lemon, Sweet Marjoram, Melissa, Myrrh, Myrtle, Niaouli, Pine, Tea Tree, Thyme.

Although Peppermint is suggested in some books, caution should be exercised as, whilst helping some individuals, it may induce pharyngeal or bronchospasm in others.

**Bronchitis:** Basil, Benzoin, Bergamot, Cajeput, Cedar, Cypress, Eucalyptus, Frankincense, Lavender, Lemon, Sweet Marjoram, Spanish Marjoram, Myrrh, Myrtle, Niaouli, Peppermint, Pine, Rosemary, Sandalwood, Thyme.

**Catarrh:** Benzoin, Cajeput, Cedar, Eucalyptus, Frankincense, Ginger, Jasmine, Lavender, Lemon, Lime, Myrrh, Myrtle, Niaouli, Black Pepper, Peppermint, Pine, Sandalwood, Tea Tree, Thyme.

**Colds and flus:** Achillea, Basil, Bergamot, Black Pepper, Cajeput, Cypress, Eucalyptus, Ginger, Grapefruit, Juniper, Lemon, Sweet Marjoram, Melissa, Myrtle, Niaouli, Peppermint, Pine, Rosemary, Tea Tree, Thyme.

**Cough:** Basil, Benzoin, Cedar, Cypress, Eucalyptus, Frankincense, Jasmine, Sweet Marjoram, Myrrh, Myrtle, Niaouli, Pine, Sandalwood, Clary Sage, Tea Tree.

**Earache:** Basil, Chamomile, Eucalyptus, Lavender, Tea Tree.

Never put neat essential oil into the ear. Either dilute at 1% total in Olive oil or macerated Verbascum oil and carefully drip 3–4 drops into the ear or place a single drop on a piece of cotton wool and place just into the ear. Warm compresses may also help.

**Gum infections/gingivitis:** Chamomile, Clove, Geranium, Myrrh, Tea Tree, Thyme.

Dilute the oils in vegetable oil and massage gums or make a mouth wash with vodka or cider vinegar (3% essential oil, dilute in teaspoon full in warm water and gargle or wash out the mouth. Aromatic salt can be made by adding the oils to sea salt and dissolving in warm water).

**Halitosis:** Bergamot, Fennel, Geranium, Lavender, Myrrh, Peppermint.

**Hayfever:** Chamomile, Eucalyptus citriodora, Juniper, Lavender, Melissa, Rose.

Use in steam inhalations. Hydrolats of Rose, Elder flower and Chamomile may also be used in cotton wool compresses to sooth eye irritation. Alternatively cold, infused Chamomile tea bags may also be used as eye packs.

**Laryngitis/loss of voice:** Benzoin, Frankincense, Jasmine, Lavender, Myrrh, Clary Sage, Sandalwood, Cypress, Thyme.

Make a gargle using glycerine or honey and tinctures of Myrrh, Calendula, Sage, Clove or other suitable herbs and add the oils.

**Mouth ulcers:** Bergamot, Eucalyptus, Geranium, Myrrh, Tea Tree.

One drop of neat essential oil can be applied with a cotton bud. Alternatively make up a mouth wash.

**Sinusitis:** Basil, Cajeput, Eucalyptus, Ginger, Lavender, Niaouli, Peppermint, Pine, Rosemary, Tea Tree.

**Sore throat:** Bergamot, Clary Sage, Eucalyptus, Geranium, Ginger, Lavender, Myrrh, Niaouli, Pine, Sandalwood, Tea Tree.

A drop of essential oil can be mixed into a teaspoonful of honey and dissolved in warm water as a gargle. Alternatively, two teaspoons of Thyme or Sage herb may be infused in a cup of boiling water. A teaspoon of honey may be added and the mixture used as a gargle when cool enough.

**Tonsillitis:** Bergamot, Geranium, Clary Sage, Lavender, Thyme, Tea Tree.

**Whooping cough:** Basil, Clary Sage, Cypress, Lavender, Rosemary, Tea Tree.

Diffusers and steam inhalations are the best forms of application.

**Loss of sense of smell:** Rosemary oil has the reputation of helping restoration of the sense of smell. I have seen this work when used in conjunction with Eucalyptus, and Peppermint.

## The skin

**Acne vulgaris, spots, pimples:** Bergamot, German Chamomile, Cedar, Geranium, Grapefruit, Immortelle, Juniper, Lavender, Lemon, Lemongrass, Mandarin, Niaouli, Palmarosa, Patchouli, Peppermint, Petitgrain, Rosemary, Clary Sage, Sandalwood, Tea Tree, Thyme, Vetivert. Compresses, face packs, lotions, creams, steaming.

**Baldness:** Bay, Cedarwood, Ginger, Juniper, Lavender, Clary Sage, Rosemary, Ylang Ylang.

Oil massage of scalp.

**Cracked and chapped skin:** Benzoin, German chamomile, Myrrh, Patchouli, Sandalwood. Calendula and German Chamomile macerated oils.

Salves and creams.

**Dandruff:** Bergamot, Cedar, Chamomile, Geranium, Juniper, Lavender, Patchouli, Peppermint, Rosemary, Clary Sage, Thyme.

Scalp massage, shampoo, conditioner.

**Dehydrated skin:** Benzoin, Chamomile, Geranium, Lavender, Neroli, Rose, Sandalwood. Also, floral waters.

Face packs, steaming, spritzes, creams.

**Dermatitis:** Benzoin, German Chamomile, Roman Chamomile, Carrot seed, Cedarwood, Immortelle, Geranium, Juniper, Lavender, Myrrh, Myrtle, Neroli, Niaouli, Palmarosa, Patchouli, Peppermint, Rose, Rosemary, Thyme linalool/geraniol.

Aromatic waters, compresses and creams, rather than oils or salves due to hot nature of condition.

**Dry Skin:** Benzoin, German Chamomile, Clary Sage, Frankincense, Geranium, Jasmine, Lavender, Myrrh, Neroli, Patchouli, Rose, Sandalwood, Vetivert.

Almond oil, Avocado oil, Jojoba oil, Shea butter, Cocoa butter. Floral waters.

**Eczema:** Bergamot, Roman and German Chamomile, Cedarwood, Geranium, Juniper, Lavender, Melissa, Myrrh, Patchouli, Rose, Rosemary, Thyme.

Compresses and creams. No oils or salves due to hot nature of condition.

**Oily skin/Hair:** Bergamot, Cedarwood, Clary Sage, Cypress, Fennel, Geranium, Jasmine, Juniper, Lavender, Lemon, Lemongrass, Mandarin, Niaouli, Patchouli, Petitgrain, Rosemary, Clary Sage, Sandalwood, Tea Tree, Vetivert, Ylang Ylang.

Hazelnut oil, Jojoba oil.

**Seborrhea:** Bergamot, German chamomile, Geranium, Frankincense, Lavender, Myrrh, Niaouli, Palmarosa, Tea tree, Thyme ct linalool or geraniol.

**Sensitive skin:** Chamomile, Neroli, Rose Otto, Sesame oil and honey.

**Thread veins:** German Chamomile, Cypress, Immortelle, Lavender, Neroli, Rose, Rosemary. Witch Hazel water, Calendula cream. Rosehip oil. Avoid steaming.

**Wrinkles/mature skin:** Carrot seed, Fennel, Frankincense, Geranium, Immortelle, Jasmine, Lavender, Mandarin, Myrrh, Neroli, Patchouli, Rose, Rosemary, Clary Sage, Sandalwood, Ylang Ylang. Also Avocado, Jojoba and Wheatgerm base oils.

**Athlete's Foot:** Cinnamon, Clove, Eucalyptus, Garlic, Geranium, Lavender, Lemon, Lemongrass, Myrrh, Oregano, Palmarosa, Patchouli, Tea Tree, Thymes.

**Boils, abscesses:** Bergamot, Chamomile, Eucalyptus, Lavender, Lemon, Clary Sage, Tea Tree, Thyme.

**Bruises:** Fennel, Geranium, Immortelle, Marjoram, Lavender, Thyme.

**Burns:** Chamomile, Eucalyptus, Geranium, Lavender, Tea Tree, Rosemary.

**Chapped skin:** Benzoin, Myrrh, Patchouli, Sandalwood.

**Chilblains:** Eucalyptus, Geranium, Lemon, Sweet Marjoram, Black Pepper.

**Cold sores/Herpes/Shingles:** Bergamot, Eucalyptus, Tea Tree. Calendula, Hypericum, Echinacea, or Melissa tincture.

**Excessive perspiration:** Cypress, Lemongrass, Pine, Clary Sage.

**Haemorrhoids/piles:** Cypress Geranium, Frankincense, Juniper, Myrrh.

**Lice:** Eucalyptus, Geranium, Lavender, Peppermint, Pine, Rosemary, Thyme.

**Scars and stretch marks:** Frankincense, Lavender, Mandarin, Neroli, Patchouli, Sandalwood.

**Varicose veins:** Cypress, Lemon, Neroli, Rose. Also Witch Hazel and Calendula compresses.

**Verrucae/warts:** Cinnamon, Lemon, Tea Tree, Tagetes.

## Muscles and bones

**Aches and Pains:** Cajeput, Chamomile, Eucalyptus, Ginger, Lavender, Lemongrass, Sweet Marjoram, Niaouli, Peppermint (only on localised areas!), Black Pepper, Pine, Rosemary, Thyme, Vetivert.

**Elimination of wastes and toxins:** Fennel, Grapefruit, Geranium, Juniper, Lemon, Mandarin, Orange, Patchouli, Black Pepper, Rosemary.

**Arthritis:** Benzoin, Cajeput, Cedarwood, Chamomile, Eucalyptus (particularly *E. citriodora*), Ginger, Juniper, Lemon, Sweet Marjoram, Myrrh, Black Pepper, Pine, Rosemary, Thyme, Vetivert. Hamamelis cream with Lemon, Birch, Cypress, Juniper.

**Gout:** Basil, Benzoin, Fennel, Juniper, Rosemary, Pine, Thyme, Geranium, Lemon.

**Rheumatism:** Basil, Benzoin, Cajeput, Chamomile, Cedar, Cypress, Eucalyptus, Fennel, Geranium, Ginger, Juniper, Lavender, Lemon, Sweet Marjoram, Niaouli, Black pepper, Pine, Rosemary, Clary Sage.

**Poor muscle tone:** Ginger, Grapefruit, Sweet Marjoram, Black Pepper, Rosemary, Pine.

**Muscle cramps and stiffness:** Cypress, Grapefruit, Jasmine, Juniper, Lavender, Lemongrass, Sweet Marjoram, Black Pepper, Pine, Rosemary, Thyme, Vetivert.

**Sprains and strains:** Chamomile, Ginger, Lavender, Sweet Marjoram, Black Pepper, Pine, Rosemary, Thyme, Vetivert.

## The digestive system

**Loss of Appetite:** Bergamot, Chamomiles, Fennel, Ginger, Black Pepper.

**Colic:** Benzoin, Bergamot, Black Pepper, Chamomile, Clary Sage, Fennel, Ginger, Juniper, Lavender, Sweet Marjoram, Peppermint, Rosemary.

**Colitis:** Black Pepper, Bergamot, Chamomile, Lavender, Neroli, Rosemary, Ylang Ylang.

**Constipation:** Black Pepper, Fennel, Ginger, Mandarin, Sweet Marjoram, Rose.

**Cramp/Gastric Spasm:** Basil, Clary Sage, Ginger, Lavender, Mandarin, Neroli, Orange, Peppermint.

**Diarrhoea:** Chamomile, Cypress, Eucalyptus, Geranium, Lavender, Myrrh, Neroli, Peppermint, Rosemary, Sandalwood.

**Flatulence:** Bergamot, Black Pepper, Chamomile, Clary Sage, Fennel, Juniper, Lavender, Sweet Marjoram, Peppermint, Rosemary.

**Gall bladder excess bile:** Rose, Rosemary. Stones—Bergamot, Eucalyptus, Lavender, Peppermint, Rosemary.

**Gastritis:** Chamomile.

**Indigestion:** Basil, Bergamot, Black Pepper, Chamomile, Clary Sage, Eucalyptus, Fennel, Frankincense, Juniper, Lavender, Sweet Marjoram, Myrrh, Peppermint, Rosemary.

**Liver congestion:** Chamomile, Cypress, Geranium, Lavender, Rose, Rosemary.

**Obesity:** Fennel, Juniper, Patchouli.

**Teething:** Chamomile, Lavender.

A 1% total dilution of these oils can be rubbed into the cheeks of babies and infants up to five. In older children, a 3% dilution can be used. In adults a drop of neat Chamomile can be massaged over the cheek and jaw. Warm compresses may also help.

**Tinnitus:** Lavender, Peppermint, and Sandalwood are reputed to help.

**Toothache:** Chamomile, Clove, Peppermint, Tea tree.

**Vomiting and Nausea:** Basil, Black Pepper, Chamomile, Fennel, Ginger, Lavender, Peppermint, Sandalwood.


*Vascular and lymphatic systems*

**Cellulite:** Cypress, Fennel, Geranium, Grapefruit, Lemon, Mandarin, Sweet Marjoram, Orange, Patchouli, Black Pepper, Pine, Rosemary.

**Hypertension:** Clary Sage, Lavender, Lemon, Sweet Marjoram, Ylang Ylang.

**Hypotension and poor circulation:** Cypress, Eucalyptus, Geranium, Ginger, Lemon, Lemongrass, Neroli, Black Pepper, Pine, Rose, Rosemary, Thyme.

**Oedema and water retention:** Cypress, Fennel, Geranium, Grapefruit, Juniper, Lemon, Mandarin, Orange, Patchouli, Rosemary.

**To constrict/tone blood vessels:** Chamomile, Cypress, Geranium, Peppermint.

**To dilate blood vessels:** Sweet Marjoram.

**Anaemia:** Grapefruit, Lemon, Soft Thyme.

## Immune function

**Adrenal cortex modulators:** Basil, Geranium, Pine, Rosemary.

**Antifungal:** Lavender, Lemongrass, Myrrh, Palmarosa, Tea Tree.

**Antiviral:** Garlic, Lavender, Tea Tree.

**Bactericide:** Most oils have some bactericidal action.

**Immunomodulants:** Clary Sage. Lavender, Tea tree, Rosemary, Sandalwood, Thyme.

**Fumigants:** Cinnamon, Clove, Eucalyptus, Lemon.

**Herpes zoster:** Pelargonium, Ravensara.

**Allergies:** Although some people do have allergic reactions to essential oils, often an individual is reacting to a rectified or adulterated oil. However, if a person has become sensitised by other factors, they may get a reaction. It is therefore a good idea to carry out patch testing on sensitive individuals. In order to relieve allergic symptoms, the following oils may be tried, bearing in mind that low dilutions should be used:

Chamomile, Juniper, Lavender, Lemon Balm, Rose.

## The reproductive and urinary systems

**Amenorrhoea/lack of menstruation:** Fennel, Juniper, Sweet Marjoram, Myrrh, Rose, Clary Sage. If there is any chance of pregnancy, essential oils should be avoided until this is confirmed.

**Bed wetting:** Chamomile, Cypress, Lavender.

**Breast engorgement:** Peppermint. Cabbage leaf compresses, or raw potato poultices. Also, Comfrey leaf and Calendula compresses.

**Cracked nipples:** Calendula ointment, Mother's milk, Wheatgerm oil.

**Cystitis:** Bergamot, Cedarwood, Chamomile, Eucalyptus, Frankincense, Juniper, Lavender, Myrtle, Pine, Sandalwood, Tea Tree, Thyme.

**Dysmenorrhoea/painful periods:** Basil, Chamomile, Cypress, Frankincense, Jasmine, Juniper, Lavender, Sweet Marjoram, Rose, Rosemary, Clary Sage.

**Hot flushes/menopause:** Chamomile, Clary Sage, Cypress, Fennel, Geranium, Jasmine.

**Labour pain and childbirth:** Clary Sage, Jasmine, Lavender, Rose.

**Lack of milk:** Fennel.

**Leucorrhoea:** Bergamot, Cedarwood, Clary Sage, Eucalyptus, Frankincense, Lavender, Sweet Marjoram, Myrrh, Rosemary, Sandalwood, Tea Tree.

**Menorrhagia:** Chamomile, Cypress, Geranium, Rose, Pine, Rosemary.

**Morning sickness:** Ginger or Peppermint tea. Inhalations of Lavender, Peppermint or Ginger oil.

**Nappy rash:** Tea Tree, Lavender or Calendula ointment.

**PMS:** Bergamot, Chamomile, Geranium, Lavender, Sweet Marjoram, Neroli, Rose.

**Thrush:** Bergamot, Geranium, Lavender, Myrrh, Tea Tree.

**Urethritis:** Bergamot, Myrtle, Tea Tree, Juniper.

**Weaning:** Epsom salt baths, Geranium, peppermint.

# CHAPTER 12

# Essential oils and emotional health

## *Essential oils and the mind*

As well as working on a pharmacological level, essential oils affect the individual by stimulating the limbic system, and therefore cause changes directly by mood enhancement and indirectly by affecting hormone and chemical secretions in the brain. The limbic system is thought to be one of the most 'primitive' parts of the brain and governs our most basic emotional responses. On a simple level, essential oils can have the effect of invigorating, stimulating, and sedating etc. They can have very specific effects, such as clearing muddled thought processes, calming oppressive anger, or reducing obsessiveness or jealousy. Some of the 'subtle' and emotional effects described are drawn from folklore and ritual, others are derived from the physiological effects of the oils, whilst others are the observations of the author. The whole area of the spiritual and emotional effects of essential oils is a course of study in itself and therefore we will concentrate on areas which are likely to be encountered in everyday life and on the more commonly used oils.

161

## Broad classifications

Note that this refers solely to emotional effects (an oil may be mentally/ emotionally sedating and physically stimulating). Also, at different doses the effect of an oil may reverse; at low levels Rosemary can be stimulating to the mind, at higher doses it may sedate. Oils can also have seemingly opposite effects depending on the individual.

**Balancing:** Geranium, Patchouli, Vetivert.

**Euphoric:** Clary Sage, Grapefruit, Rose, Ylang Ylang.

**Sedative:** Benzoin, Bergamot, Chamomile (Roman and German), Cedarwood both, Cypress, Frankincense, Jasmine, Juniper, Lavender, Lemongrass, Mandarin, Sweet marjoram, Melissa, Myrrh, Orange, Neroli, Patchouli, Petitgrain, Sandalwood, Vetivert.

**Stimulating:** Basil, Black Pepper, Cardamom, Coriander, Eucalyptus radiata globulus and citriodora, Fennel, Ginger, Grapefruit, Lemon, Lemongrass, Lime, Peppermint, Pine, Rosemary, Thyme, Tea tree.

**Uplifting:** Bergamot, Mandarin, Melissa, Orange, Palmarosa.

**Anxiety:** Benzoin, Bergamot, Chamomile, Cedar, Cypress, Frankincense, Geranium, Jasmine, Juniper, Lavender, Sweet Marjoram, Melissa, Neroli, Patchouli, Rose, Sandalwood, Ylang ylang.

**Lack of confidence:** Jasmine, Neroli.

**Low spirits:** Basil, Bergamot, Chamomile, Clary Sage, Frankincense, Grapefruit, Geranium, Jasmine, Lavender, Melissa, Neroli, Patchouli, Rose, Sandalwood, Vetivert, Ylang Ylang.

**Fatigue and nervous exhaustion:** Basil, Cardamom, Clary Sage, Eucalyptus, Geranium, Ginger, Grapefruit, Jasmine, Lemongrass, Sweet Marjoram, Patchouli, Peppermint, Pine, Rosemary, Rosewood/ Ho Leaf, Thyme, Ti Tree, Vetivert, Ylang Ylang.

**Grief:** Benzoin, Bergamot, Chamomile, Lavender, Melissa, Neroli, Sweet Marjoram, Rose.

**Hyperactivity:** Clary Sage, Lavender, Mandarin, Sweet Marjoram, Ylang Ylang.

**Insomnia:** Basil, Benzoin, Bergamot, Chamomile, Clary Sage, Jasmine, Lavender, Mandarin, Sweet Marjoram, True Melissa, Neroli, Petitgrain, Rose, Sandalwood, Vetivert, Ylang Ylang.

**Irritability:** Chamomile, Frankincense, Geranium, Grapefruit, Lavender, Neroli, Rose, Sandalwood, Ylang Ylang.

**Memory Stimulants:** Basil, Grapefruit, Lemon, Peppermint, Rosemary.

**Migraine And Headaches:** Basil, Chamomile, Clary Sage (Unless It Nauseates), Lavender, Sweet Marjoram, Melissa, Peppermint.

**Palpitations:** Chamomile, Lavender, Neroli, Rose, Ylang Ylang.

**Shock:** Lavender, Melissa, Neroli, Peppermint.

**Exam nerves:** Bergamot, Lavender, Neroli, Peppermint, Rosemary, Ylang Ylang.

**Stress:** Most essential oils are good for stress!!

Even when using oils on a mental/emotional level, it is a good idea to change the blend regularly. This is partly to keep up with changes in your psyche.

# CHAPTER 13

# Formulations for various conditions

Some tried and tested formulae that have proved valuable in practice. These are formulae that I have used regularly but they can also be used as suggestions that can be adapted for individual patients, since we treat the person as an individual. It is better to individualise the treatment for the person rather than just be treating a condition without considering them as a whole.

*Integumentary system*

**Wounds:**
Lavender 1 ml
Geranium 1 ml
Tea tree 1 ml
Rosemary (preferably verbenone CT) 1 ml
Immortelle 5 gtt
Tamanu 5 ml
Rosehip 5 ml
Calendula-infused oil 20 ml
German Chamomile 5 drops

St John's Wort infused oil 20 ml
Apply to wound on gauze or lint and refresh every twelve hours.

**Puncture wounds (antiseptic blend):**
Tea tree 1 ml
Peppermint 5 drops
Lavender 1 ml
Thyme 4 drops
   Five drops onto some cotton wool; renew every 6–12 hours.
Capsicum tincture is also an option.

**Bruises:**
50/50 blend Comfrey and Arnica/Daisy cream
1% each Immortelle, Geranium, German Chamomile, Sweet Marjoram,
   Lavender.

**Burns:**
Cool area under running water or with ice. Apply neat Lavender or
Lavandin oil. A drop of Peppermint can be added to help reduce pain.
Repeat every couple of hours. German Chamomile can also be used,
either using the tea bags as compresses (cool in this case) or the oil
diluted to about 5%. Alternatively, 1:5 Immortelle, Tamanu applied 4–6
times daily.

**Scars, prevention and reduction of older ones:**
50/50 Rosehip oil and Avocado oil
2% Immortelle, 2% Frankincense or Mandarin, 1% Neroli or Petitgrain

**Shingles:**
10 ml Tea Tree
1 ml Geranium
5 ml *Eucalyptus smithii*
1 ml *Eucalyptus citriodora* or other aldehyde-rich oil
0.5 ml Peppermint as analgesic and antiviral
   This blend can be diluted with St John's Wort oil or tincture before
application.

**Bacterial skin infections:**
Thyme (thujanol)
Tea Tree

Eucalyptus (*E. globulus*)
Palmarosa
Up to 5% of each in a base lotion/gel/cream.

Internally use one drop each of Thyme thujanol, Palmarosa, and Tea Tree in a teaspoonful of vegetable oil three times daily or suitable tincture formula.

**Fungal skin infections (and nail infections):**
1% Cinnamon
5% Tea Tree
1% Geranium
1% Oregano
In Neem oil base.

Apply twice daily for three weeks and then review; if necessary switch to alcohol-rich oil formula above then back to this.

**Thread veins:**
50 ml Rosehip oil
10 ml German chamomile
10 ml Lavender
10 ml Geranium

Apply the blend twice daily over the affected area.

**Varicose veins:**
50:50 Calendula, Witch Hazel cream
1% each Cypress, Rosemary, Geranium, Lemon
0.5% German Chamomile, Frankincense, Patchouli, Sandalwood.

Apply two to three times daily over the affected veins.

**Lipoma:**
Base cream 1% each Geranium, Lemon, and Eucalyptus (*Eucalyptus citriodora* and *globulus*).

Apply twice daily over the lipoma.

**Warts/verrucae:**
1 part Cinnamon
4 parts Tea Tree
5 parts Lemon

Apply to affected area twice daily until they are clear. For verrucae a corn plaster (the ones with a hole in the middle) can be valuable, since it relieves pressure (and they thrive on this) and helps to ensure that the oils are only applied to the affected area.

## Respiratory system

For acute respiratory infections, or indeed long-term support of the lungs, I favour applications via the soles of the feet. The circulation returns the oils pretty directly up to the lungs, bypassing the portal circulation and the oils are excreted through the lungs, effecting treatment on their way out. Also the reflexes for the lungs are in this area. The treatment may be enhanced by also applying a salve or oil blend between the shoulders or over the clavicle and using steam inhalations.

It may be useful to treat in several stages as follows:

1. Mucolytic 2 days eg

    15 ml *Eucalyptus smithii*
    5 ml *Picea mariana* Black Spruce
    1 ml *Mentha spicata*

Or

    15 ml *Eucalyptus smithii*
    4 ml *Pinus sylvestris* Scots Pine
    1 ml *Eucalyptus globulus*

2. Infection treatment
3. Convalescence—specifically supporting immune system and liver.

I tend to go for mucolysis, infection treatment, and immune support at the same time; for example:
4 ml Lavender/Lavandin *L. vera* or *x intermedia*
4 ml Eucalyptus (*E. globulus* or *smithii*)
2 ml Pine/Spruce (*Pinus sylvestris/Picea mariana*)

Bear in mind the basic precept that we are balancing the 'terrain' rather than waging war on an invading pathogen.

### Viral infections

Thyme (linalool; *Thymus vulgaris* ct. linalol), Myrtle (*Myrtus communis*), Eucalyptus (*E. smithii*, or *E. globulus* if patient is over twelve years old),

Tea Tree (*Melaleuca alternifolia*), Frankincense (*Boswellia carterii*), Sandalwood (*Santalum album*), Pine (*Pinus sylvestris*).

**Bacterial infections**

Tea Tree (*Melaleuca alternifolia*)/Ravensara (*Ravensara aromatica*), Myrtle (*Myrtus communis*), Pine (*Pinus sylvestris*), Eucalyptus (*E. smithii* or *globulus*), Oregano (*Origanum vulgare*), Cinnamon (*Cinnamomum verum*), Thyme (*Thymus vulgaris*), Rosemary (*Rosmarinus officinalis*).

For example:

15 ml *Eucalyptus smithii*
3 ml Myrtle (*Mytrus communis*)
1 ml Rosemary (*Rosmarinus officinalis*)
1 ml *Eucalyptus globulus*

Warm the feet with a hair drier. If particularly acute, start with 10–20 drops on each foot every fifteen minutes and then gradually reduce to every hour, then every two hours then three times a day.

**Colds/rhinovirus**

A combination of steam inhalations or inhalations from a tissue and frictions over the occipital ridge and down the lymph gland chains of the throat is extremely effective. Friction every two hours and steam twice in the day.

- Inhalation blend:

1 drop each of Eucalyptus (*E. globulus/smithii/radiata*), Tea Tree/Ravensara, Lavender in a bowl of boiling water. Inhale deeply through nose for 5–15 minutes.

- Friction blend:

2 *Eucalyptus globulus/smithii*
1 Rosemary (*Rosmarinus officinalis*)
1 Ginger (*Zingiber officinale*)
5 Tea Tree (*Melaleuca alternifolia*)
1 Frankincense (*Boswellia carterii*)
2 Lavender (*Lavandula vera*)
1 Peppermint (*Mentha x piperita*)
1 Thyme (*Thymus vulgaris*) (linalool)

1 Pine (*Pinus sylvestris*)
Rub 5–10 drops over the occiput and lymph chains every two hours.

### Bronchiolitis
3 Eucalyptus (*E. smithii*)
2 Myrtle (*Myrtus communis*)
2 Lavender (*Lavandula vera*)
1 Thyme (*Thymus vulgaris*) (linalool)
1 Sandalwood (*Santalum album*)
1 Spruce (*Picea mariana*)
Mix at 10% in a base oil and apply liberally to the feet every two hours initially and then reduce to three times a day.

### Emphysema
Inhalations of equal parts Cypress (*Cupressus sempervirens*), Pine (*Pinus sylvestris*), and Black Spruce (*Picea mariana*).
The blend can also be diluted to 5% and massaged over the thorax.

### Sinusitis
Use inhalations and frictions; compresses or poultices (face packs) can also benefit. The formula will vary depending on whether there is infection present but in general it is good to include some bacteriostatic oils to help prevent an infection occurring. Also, consider whether it is a hot or cold condition and treat accordingly.

Hot—*Eucalyptus citirodora*, Lavender (*Lavandula vera*), German Chamomile (*Matricaria recutita*), Peppermint (*Mentha x piperita*), Pine (*Pinus sylvestris*).

Cold—Rosemary (*Rosmarinus officinalis*), Peppermint (*Mentha x piperita*), Eucalyptus (any species), Lavender (*Lavandula vera*), Pine (*Pinus sylvestris*), Tea Tree (*Melaleuca alternifolia*).

### Ear Infections
Although oils can be put neat onto cotton wool and placed into the ear, I prefer to make a blend that is massaged behind the auricula/pinna. This is easy to repeat every couple of hours. The absorption of the oils can be facilitated with a hot pack (hot water bottle) and this also eases the pain.

Verbascum macerated oil

1 part Lavender (*Lavandula vera*)

1 part German Chamomile (*Matricaria recutita*)

2 parts Tea tree (*Melaleuca alternifolia*)

1 part Thyme (*Thymus vulgaris*) (thujanol) (if not available use Geranium (*Pelargonium graveolens*) or Palmarosa (*Cymbopogon martini*))

### Acute earache/ear infection in a child

1 ml Tea tree (*Melealeuca alternifolia*)

1.5 ml Niaouli (*M. quinquinervia*)

1 ml Lavender (*Lavandula vera*)

0.5 ml Thyme (*Thymus vulgaris*) ct linalool

Macerated oil of Calendula/Verbascum/Hypericum.

Rub around the ear as described above

### Chronic Earache and Serous Otitis

The catarrh comes from the nose and therefore steaming will also help. As will washing with a Neti pot. Apply a friction of the formula below to the lymph nodes in the neck and along the occipital ridge 2–4 times daily.

2 ml Tea Tree (*Melaleuca alternifolia*)

1 ml Myrtle (*Myrtus communis*)

1 ml Lavender (*Lavandula vera*)

2 ml Wild Marjoram (*Thymus mastichina*)

10 ml Tamanu (*Caulophyllum inophyllum*)

14 ml Calendula or Hypericum macerated oil

### Hay Fever/Allergic Rhinitis

Inhalations with Myrtle (*Myrtus communis*), German Chamomile (*Matricaria recutia*), *Eucalyptus citriodora, Eucalyptus globulus/smithii* are helpful since they help ease the inflammation, but also flush out any irritant particles.

### Cold Sores

Tincture of Calendula (90% alcohol one), Hypericum or Melissa or equal parts of all three. To this add:

5% Tea tree (*Melaleuca alternifolia*)

4% *Eucalyptus globulus/smithii*
1% Lemon
(*Citrus limomum*)

## Digestive system

### Motion Sickness
A single drop of Peppermint (*Mentha x piperita*) oil. Not suitable for children under twelve—in this case place a drop on a tissue for them to inhale. Alternatively, use Ginger tea or sucking a piece of crystallized Ginger.

### Digestive Tonic
1 ml Peppermint (*Mentha x piperita*)
2 ml Dill (*Anethum graveolens*)
3 ml Tarragon (*Artemisia dranculus*)
1 ml Black pepper (*Piper nigrum*)
    Add 1–3 drops to a teaspoon of honey and dissolve in warm water. Alternatively, dilute to 3% in a carrier oil and massage over the abdomen.

## Musculoskeletal system

### Arthritis
10 ml Tea Tree (*Melaleuca alternifolia*)
5 ml Rosemary (*Rosmarinus officinalis*)
5 ml Lavandin (*Lavandula x intermedia*)
1 ml Ginger (*Zingiber officinale*)
1 ml Black Pepper (*Piper nigrum*)
1 ml Nutmeg (*Myristica fragrans*)
3 ml Geranium/Palmarosa (*Pelargonium graveolens/Cymbopogon martini*)
1 ml Peppermint (*Mentha x piperita*)
1 ml Eucalyptus (*E. citriodora*)
1 ml Cinnamon (*Cinnamomum verum*)
    Either use a few drops neat for small area of application or dilute to 5% in carrier for larger area.

### Tendonitis
Tamanu base with 0.5% Birch and 1% Eucalyptus (*E. citriodora*).

### Gout
4 ml Tea Tree/Niaouli (*Melaleuca alternifolia/M. quinquinervia*)
1 ml Peppermint (*Mentha x piperita*)

2 ml Lemon (*Citrus limonum*)
1 ml Juniper (*Juniperus communis*)
2 m Geranium (*Pelargonium graveolens*)
  Dilute to 10% in a Comfrey cream and apply liberally to affected area as needed to reduce pain (up to six times a day)

## Urinary system

**Acute Cystitis**
Tea Tree (*Melaleuca alternifolia*), Soft Thyme (*Thymus vulgaris*), Bergamot (*Citrus bergamia*) equal parts diluted to 3% in a carrier cream and applied liberally over the lower back and pubic area, 3–5 times daily.

**Balanitis:**
60 g Chamomile or Calendula cream
12 drops Ravensara (*Ravensara aromatica*)
12 drops German Chamomile (*Matricaria recutita*)
12 drops Lavender (*Lavandula vera*)
  Apply up to five times daily.

## Lymphatic system

*Lymphatic Absorption Cream Formula*
In a base cream use up to 10%:
4% Tea tree (*Melaleuca alternifolia*)
2% Niaouli (*M. quinquinervia*)
1% Geranium (*Pelargonium graveolens*)
1% Rosemary (*Rosmarinus officinalis*)
2% Lemon or Grapefruit (*C.limomum/medica*)
  Apply 3–6 times daily to congested lymph nodes or to the lymph nodes nearest to the area that you wish to drain/clean. This can be combined with dry skin brushing, rebounding, massage, stimulation of the lymphatic reflexes, and many other techniques to get things moving.

## Gynaecological conditions

Neat oils soaked into a tampon are not an option. It is possible to dilute essential oils in yogurt or a carrier oil and syringe them into the vagina, but this is a little messy and many people just are not able to do this every couple of hours in their normal routine. I compromise by making up an absorption cream which can be applied over the pubis and sacrum every two hours and this seems to work.

Hydrosols can be valuable for use as douches or 'vaginal injections'.

## Thrush
Cream base—Calendula, Chamomile, or plain base cream
1 part Geranium/Palmarosa (*Pelargonium graveolens/Cymbopogon martini*)
2 parts Tea Tree/Ravensara (*Melaleuca alternifolia/Ravensara aromatica*)
1 part German Chamomile (*Matricaria recutita*)
1 part Lemongrass (*Cymbopogon nardus*)/Eucalyptus (*E. citriodora*)
1 part Lavender (*Lavandula vera*)/Soft Thyme (*Thymus vulgaris*)
1 part Cinnamon (*Cinnamomum verum*)
2 parts Eucalyptus (*E. globulus*)
1 part Myrrh (*Commiphora molmol*)
Alternatively:
4 parts Tea tree (*Melaleuca alternifolia*)
2 part Palmarosa (*Cymbopogon martini*)
1.5 parts Geranium (*Geranium graveolens*)
1 part Lavender (*Lavandula vera*)
1 part Thyme (*Thymus vulgaris*) thujanol
0.5 part Rosemary (*Rosmarinus officinalis*)
Dilute to 10% in a gel or lotion. This can also help with dysplasia.

## Bacterial Infections (including chlamydia)
Base cream (10%):
4 part Soft Thyme (*Thymus vulgaris*)
3 part *Eucalyptus globulus*
1 part Peppermint (*Mentha x piperita*)
1 part Oregano (*Origanum vulgare*)
1 part Ravensara/Tea Tree (*Ravensara aromatica/Melaleuca alternifolia*)

## Dysplasia
Niaouli and Eucalyptus (*E. polybractea*—crypoton type) are especially effective.

60 g base cream or macerated Calendula cream

10 drops each Geranium (*Pelargonium graveolens*), Eucalyptus (*E. polybractea*), Sandalwood (*Santalum album*), Myrtle (*Myrtus communis*), Niaouli (*Melaleuca quinquinervia*), Frankincense (*Boswellia carterii*).

**Batholinitis**
Immortelle (*Helichrysum italicum*), Rosemary verbenone (*Rosmarinus officinalis*)
Equal parts to 10% in base oil. A lower dilution may be necessary.

**Dysmennorhoea**
Use frictions of up to 5% over the abdomen and sacrum of the following oils; Sweet Marjoram (*Origanum marjorana*), Ginger (*Zingiber officinale*), Lavender (*Lavandula vera*), Roman Chamomile (*Anthemis nobilis*), Clary Sage(Salvia sclarea) (unless driving etc. due to sedative effect).

**To Facilitate Delivery**
Up to 5% Clove bud(*Eugenia caryophyllum*) or Clary Sage(*Salvia sclarea*), or 1% Jasmine (*Jasminum grandofloum/officinale*). Massage around the sacrum. Bear in mind that the senses become particularly acute during labour so the aroma may be too much. If a baby is overdue the Clove bud or Clary Sage can be used to encourage the onset of labour once there are no complications.

## *Neuroendocrine function*

**Adrenal Support**
5 parts Black Spruce or Pine (*Picea mariana/Pinus sylvestris*)
1 part Atlas Cedar (*Cedrus altlantica*)
Apply a few drops over the kidneys three times daily, or in extreme cases (or withdrawal from steroids) use every two hours.
Alternatively:
1% Geranium (*Pelargonium graveolens*)
1% Rosemary (*Rosmarinus officinalis*)
1% Pine or Spruce in a carrier oil massaged over the kidney/adrenal area 2–5 times daily

**Nervous Exhaustion**
A friction of 10 drops of Tea Tree or Ravensara (*Melaleuca alternifolia/Ravensara aromatica*) on either side of the spine followed by several hours rest can be extremely revitalising.

**Nervous Tension**
Personally, I tend to use teas, tinctures, or aromatic waters internally for this, but this can be supported by frictions of oils over the solar plexus, wrists, and temples or the use of oils in diffusers and baths.

Three examples of helpful blends are:

- Roman Chamomile (*Anthemis nobilis*), Clary Sage (*Salvai sclarea*), Mandarin (*Citrus reticulata*)
- Ylang Ylang (*Cananga odorata*), Mandarin (*Citrus reticulata*), Sweet Marjoram (*Origanum marjorana*)
- Mandarin (*Citrus reticulata*), Petitgrain (*Citrus aurantium fol.*), Lemongrass (*Cymbopogon nardus*)

Equally, three drops (total) of any of the blends could be taken in a teaspoon of vegetable oil or honey, three times daily. If Clary Sage is being taken internally avoid alcohol, driving, or operation of heavy machinery—this blend is better for night time use rather than during the day.

**Insomnia**
5 ml Lavender (*Lavandula angustifolia*)
1 ml Roman Chamomile (*Anthemis nobilis*)
1 ml German Chamomile (*Matricaria recutita*)

Or

3 ml Ylang ylang (*Cananga odorata*)
2 ml Lavender (*Lavandula vera*)
2 ml Sweet Marjoram (*Origanum marjorana*)
Take 3–5 drops, twenty minutes before bed
I either make pills or imbue the oils onto charcoal tablets to prevent damage to the digestive lining.

**Vasovagal Syncope**
This blend is used as an inhalant or can be used on a tissue to smell if knowing one is going to be be exposed to a trigger. It is also good for sinusitis. Either use the blend by inhalation or the alternative is to add at 3% to a cream to apply under the nose for vasovagal attacks or over the sinuses for sinus inflammation.
15 ml Lavandin
15 ml Eucalyptus ((*Lavandula x intermedia*)*E. globulus*)

10 ml Pine (*Pinus sylvestris*)
5 ml Peppermint (*Mentha x piperita*)
5 ml Rosemary (*Rosmarinus officinalis*)
5 ml Tea Tree(*Melaleuca laternifolia*)

## Sundry formulae

Below are some other formulae that do not fit neatly under a single system.

### Deep Tissue Healing Salve
Used for arthritis and rheumatism but also good for peripheral neuropathy, chest infections, and pleural discomfort
250 ml infused oil of Daisy (*Bellis perennis*) or Immortelle (*Helichrysum italicum*) or Arnica (*Arnica montana*)
250 ml infused oil of Comfrey leaf (*Symphytum officinale fol.*) or Ribwort Plantain (*Plantago lanceolata*)
250 ml infused oil of Marigold (*Calendula officinalis* flos.)
250 ml infused oil of St. John's Wort (*Hypericum perforatum*)
125 ml infused oil of Capsicum/Chilli
75 g beeswax
Warm these together in a bain-marie until the beeswax is melted. then add the following essential oils:

20 ml Lavandin (*Lavandula x intermedia*)
10 ml Peppermint (*Mentha x piperita*)
5 ml Ginger (*Zingiber officinale*)
5 ml Birch or Wintergreen (*Betula* sp., *Gaultheria procumbens*)—make sure this is the natural form rather than synthetic methyl salicylate
Pour into jars and allow to cool.

### Plantain and Daisy Salve
Used for bumps, bruises, bites (including horse fly), stings, sprains, and strains.
250 ml Daisy-infused oil
250 ml Plantain-infused oil
35 g beeswax

Warm in a bain marie until the beeswax is melted. Add 2% each Lavandin and Tea Tree essential oils. Pour into jars and leave to set.

**Insect Repellent**
100 ml base oil
6 gtt Lemongrass (*Cymbopogon nardus*)
3 *Eucalyptus globulus*
3 Basil (*Ocimum basilicum*)
3 Peppermint (*Mentha x piperita*)
3 Geranium (*Pelargonium graveolens*)
3 Cedar (*Cedrus atlantica*)
3 Patchouli (*Pogostemon cablin*)

You could also add some Cistus (*Cistus incanus*) oil and drink a tea. Effective against horse flies, moths (spray for clothes), and many other flying things. Possibly effective against ticks too.

# CONCLUDING REMARKS

In nearly forty years of practice, I have found essential oils to be an invaluable part of my pharmacy and therapeutic repertoire, which I highly recommend exploring.

Much of my approach has been informed by older texts written by practitioners, rather than theorists or academics; people such as Jean Valnet, Marguerite Maury, Thomas Bartram, Patricia Davis, and many others, who used these wonderful oils as part of their busy practices, and by discussions with people with extensive experience of working with the oils. There may not have been lots of peer reviewed and 'evidenced-based' information in my approach. However, it is informed by the best evidence ever—the therapeutic results obtained by these practitioners.

My choice of oils has been informed by my passion for sustainability on all levels, but especially environmental, biodiversity, and social levels. The best oils are produced by artisans who have spent many years learning their skills and who practice wildcrafting that cares for their ecosystems or what would now be called regenerative agriculture principles, which care for the environment and the soil. These artisanal skills are invaluable and produce the most amazing healing oils that allow people in rural areas to earn a fair income through their products—especially if we get them via short supply chains.

As the title of this book says, it is a concise manual of what I have found useful. It does not cover all approaches or all possibilities, but hopefully it is sufficient to enthuse people to use essential oils with confidence and with safe information.

I hope you enjoy your explorations.

# BIBLIOGRAPHY

Brand, G., & Millot, J. L. (2001). Sex differences in human olfaction: between evidence and enigma. *The Quarterly Journal of Experimental Psychology: Section B, 54*(3), 259–270.

Caddy, R. (1997). Essential Oils in Colour Great Britain: Amberwood Publishing.

Corbin, A. (1986). The Foul and the Fragrant Odour and the Social Imagination London: Macmillan.

Cytowic, R. (2003). The Man Who Tasted Shapes Massachusetts: MIT Press Ltd.

Dalton, P., Doolittle, N., & Breslin, P. A. (2002). Gender-specific induction of enhanced sensitivity to odors. *Nature Neuroscience, 5*(3), 199–200. University of Copenhagen. (2008, December 18). Girls have Superior Sense of Taste to Boys. *Science Daily*. Retrieved July 15, 2017 from www.sciencedaily.com/releases/2008/12/081216104035.htm

Davis, P. (1988). A–Z of Aromatherapy UK: C. W. Daniel Company Ltd.

Davis, P. (1991). Subtle Aromatherapy Saffron Walden: C. W. Daniel Company Ltd.

Delplanque, S., Grandjean, D., Chrea, C., Aymard, L., Cayeux, I., Le Calve, B., ... & Sander, D. (2008). Emotional processing of odors: evidence for a nonlinear relation between pleasantness and familiarity evaluations. *Chemical Senses, 33*(5), 469–479.

Franchomme, P., Penoel, D. (1995). l'aromatherapie Exactement Limoges: Roger Joillois.

Grosjean, N. (1993). Aromatherapy from Provence Saffron Walden: C. W. Daniel Company Ltd.

Gumbel, D. (1984). Principles of Holistic Therapy with Herbal Esssences Haug International Brussels Herz, R. S., & Inzlicht, M. (2002). Sex differences in response to physical and social factors involved in human mate selection: The importance of smell for women. *Evolution and Human Behavior, 23*(5), 359–364.

Kielhorn, J., Melching-Kollmub, Mangelsdorf (2006). Dermal Absorption pub. World Health Organisation.

Lautié, R., & Passebecq, A. (1984). Aromatherapy Thorsons.

Lawless, J. (1992). The Encyclopaedia of Essential Oils Shaftesbury: Element Books Ltd.

Mailhebiau, P. (1995). Portraits in Oils Saffron Walden: C. W. Daniel Company Ltd.

Peace Rhind, J. (2012). Essential oils London: Singing Dragon/Jessica Kingsley Publishers.

Price, L., & Price, S. (2007). Aromatherapy for Health Professionals Churchill Livingstone Elsevier.

Ryman, D. (1991). Aromatherapy London: Judy piatkus (Publishers) Ltd.

Schnaubelt, K. (1998). Advanced Aromatherapy Vermont: Healing Arts Press.

Schnaubelt, K. (1999). Medical Aromatherapy Berkley: Frog Press Ltd.

Sellar, W. (1992). The Directory of Essential Oils Saffron Walden: C. W. Daniel Company Ltd.

Skipper, C., & de Bonneval, P. Aromatic Medicine, Integrating essential oils into herbal practice Lyons: Éditions des Savoir Naturels.

Scheider, R., Singer, N., Singer, T. Medical aromatherapy revisited. *Human Psychopharmacology Clinical and Experimental.* 2018.

Valnet, J. (1980). The Practice of Aromatherapy Saffron Walden: C. W. Daniel Company Ltd.

Van Toller. (1999). *Chemical Senses, 24*(6), 705–712. https://doi.org/10.1093/chemse/24.6.705

Worwood, V. (1990). The Fragrant Pharmacy London: Macmillan.

# INDEX